THE
HOME APOTHECARY

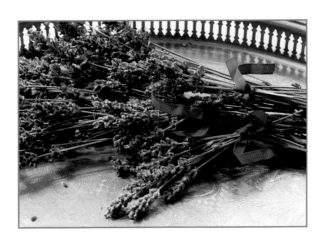

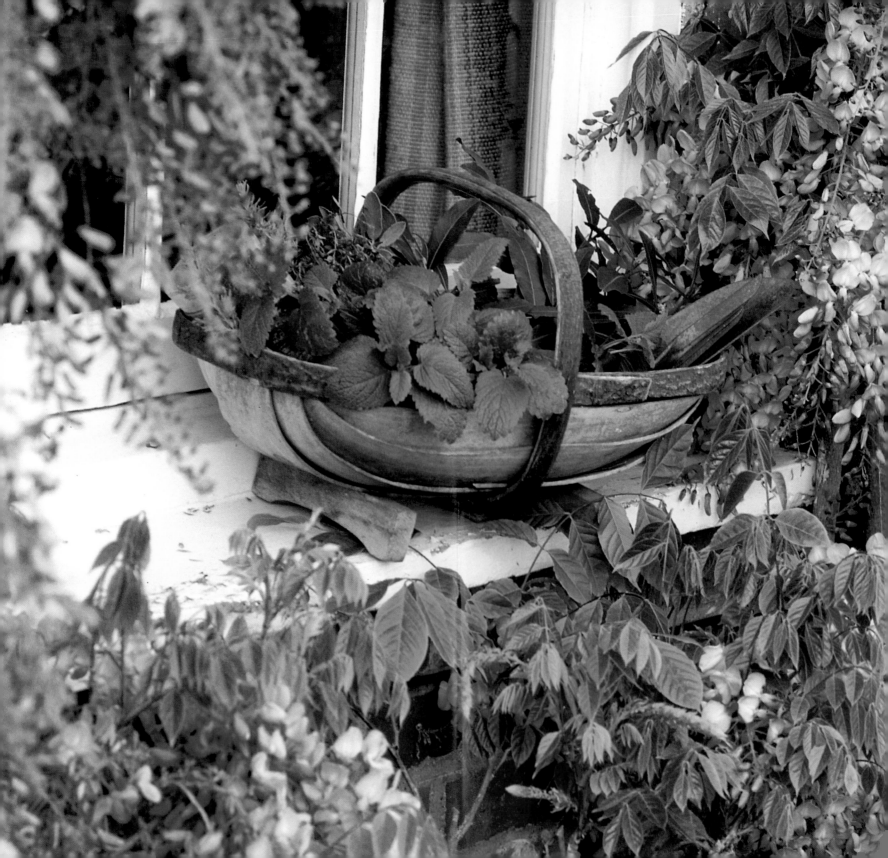

THE
HOME APOTHECARY

Jessica Houdret

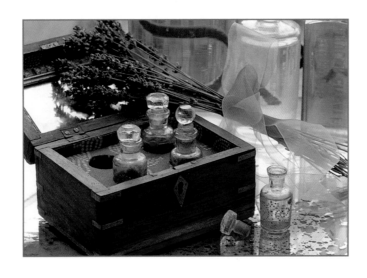

Photography by Michelle Garrett

LORENZ BOOKS

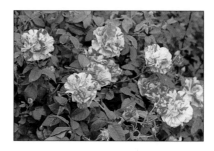

This edition first published in 1998 by Lorenz Books
27 West 20th Street, New York, NY 10011

Lorenz Books are available for bulk purchase for sales promotion and for
premium use. For details, write or call the sales director:
Lorenz Books, 27 West 20th Street, New York, NY 10011; (800) 354-9657

ISBN 1 85967 608 1

Publisher: Joanna Lorenz
Project Editor: Fiona Eaton
Designer: Nigel Partridge
Photographer: Michelle Garrett

Printed and bound in Singapore

3 5 7 9 10 8 6 4 2

—*IMPORTANT NOTICE*—

The recipes in this book have all been tried and tested, but any
plant, cosmetic or animal substance can cause allergic reactions
in certain people. Neither the author nor the publishers can be
held responsible for inappropriate use of any of the remedies or
beauty treatments, nor for excessive intake or mistaken identity
of any of the plants. Advice from a medical practitioner should
always be sought for any persistent symptom, or for any serious
or long-term condition.

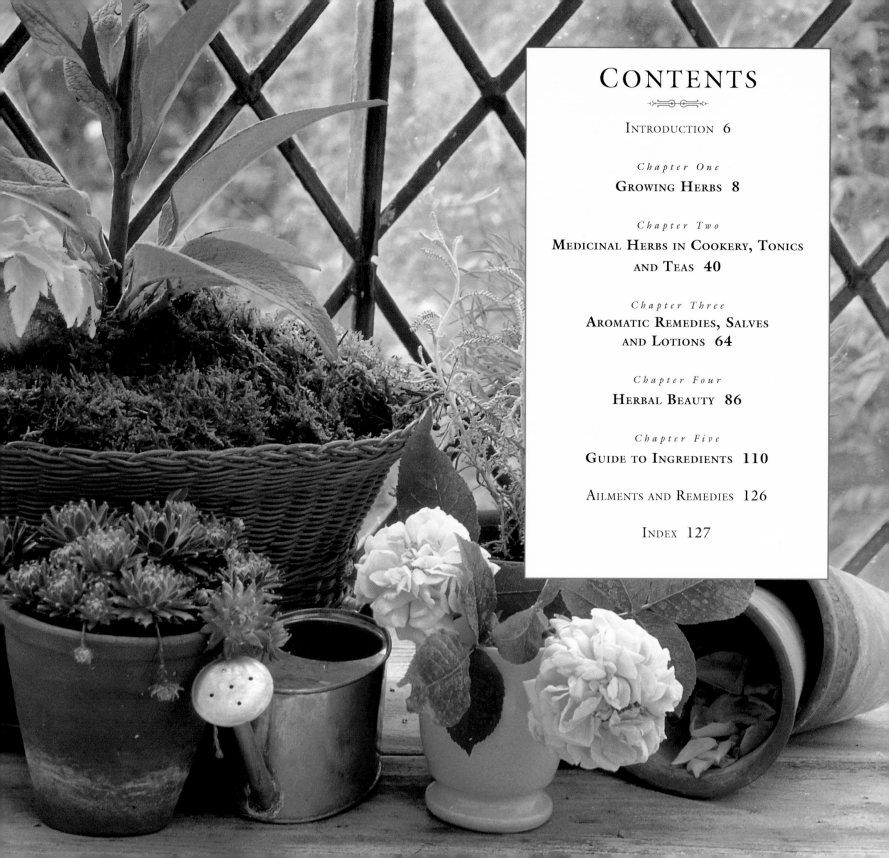

CONTENTS

INTRODUCTION 6

Chapter One
GROWING HERBS 8

Chapter Two
MEDICINAL HERBS IN COOKERY, TONICS AND TEAS 40

Chapter Three
AROMATIC REMEDIES, SALVES AND LOTIONS 64

Chapter Four
HERBAL BEAUTY 86

Chapter Five
GUIDE TO INGREDIENTS 110

AILMENTS AND REMEDIES 126

INDEX 127

INTRODUCTION

The apothecary of medieval England prepared and traded medicines made from exotic spices, resins and aromatics, imported from the East, and from the humble plants of the countryside. Most apothecaries kept their own physic gardens so as to have the right plants to hand. They also bought or collected from the wild "simples" – individual medicinal plants – from which they concocted their "compounds".

There was a universal belief in the power of fragrance to protect from disease, which led to the production of pomanders, the use of posies,

BELOW: Pomanders can be made of scented resin or spice-studded apples and oranges.

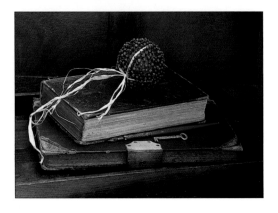

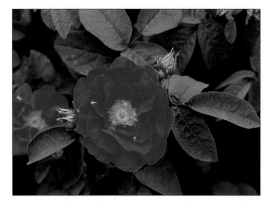

ABOVE: The Apothecary's Rose, Rosa gallica officinalis, was an important medicinal herb.

strewing herbs and herbal fumigation. Diet was also considered integral to healing – herbs and flowers were added to food for their medicinal action as much as for their nutritional or flavouring capabilities.

When making their remedies, the apothecaries were guided by the herbals: the earliest of which was written in China, nearly 5,000 years ago, but because China remained closed to the West for many centuries, it is the herbal texts recorded on tablets and papyri from the early civilizations of Sumeria and Egypt which are the antecedents of the later European herbals. The great physicians of ancient Greece – Hippocrates, Galen, Theophrastus and Dioscorides – drew on these earlier cultures when writing their own works. Their texts were kept alive through the Dark Ages, copied by successive generations of monks, and given a new lease of life with the discovery of printing in the mid-fifteenth century. Dioscorides' *De Materia Medica* formed the basis of many of the early printed European herbals.

In the sixteenth century, European herbalists took a new line in their work, based on empirical observations of plants. John Gerard's *Herball and General History of Plants*, in this tradition of enquiry, was first published in England in 1597. The great age of the medical herbals was coming to an end by the time John Parkinson published his *Theatrum Botanicum* in 1650, when Nicholas Culpeper's *English Physician* also appeared.

The role of the apothecaries was changing. At the beginning of the sixteenth century, they had established their own society and were the pharmacists of the time, dispensing drugs for the physicians and giving medical advice to patients. By the following century, membership of the Society of Apothecaries was restricted to medical practitioners, and in 1815 it was granted powers to examine and license all who practised medicine. The apothecary had made the final transition to general practitioner.

This transition coincided with the rise of modern scientific enquiry, and the medical establishment turned away from remedies made with plants to laboratory-produced chemical drugs. This was a great step forward for civilization as general health improved, life expectancy increased and cures were found for many diseases, but the side-effect was that much of the responsibility for their own minor health problems was taken out of the hands of

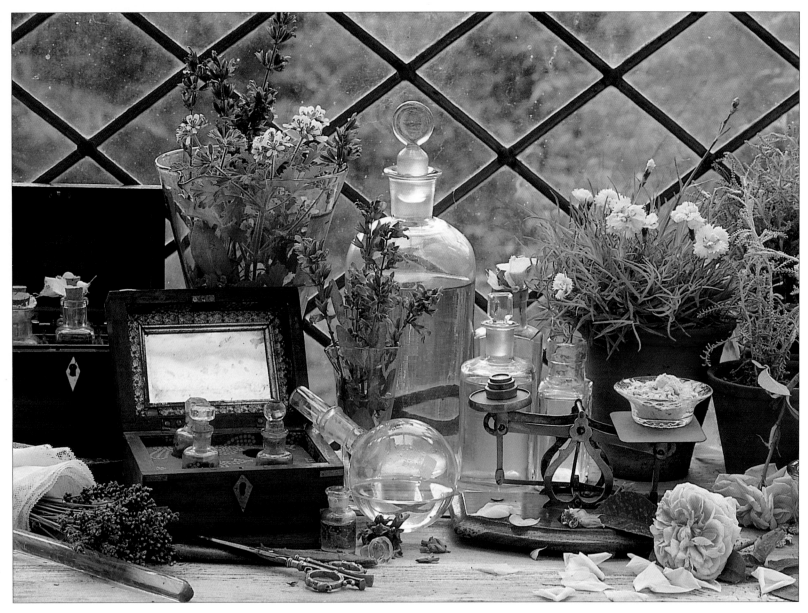

ABOVE: Medicinal and aromatic compounds were concocted in the still-rooms of houses.

ordinary people and simple home remedies were forgotten. However, much of this ancient plant lore has since been vindicated by modern research, which has established that many herbs have antibacterial, antifungal and other medicinal properties.

This book contains easy plant-based recipes for treating everyday ailments, along with a number of beauty recipes that are beneficial to general health and well-being. The power of fragrance is also recognized, if not to ward off infection, at least to alter mood and state of mind. There is also a section on using herbs and spices in the diet and advice on growing herbs as raw materials for the remedies.

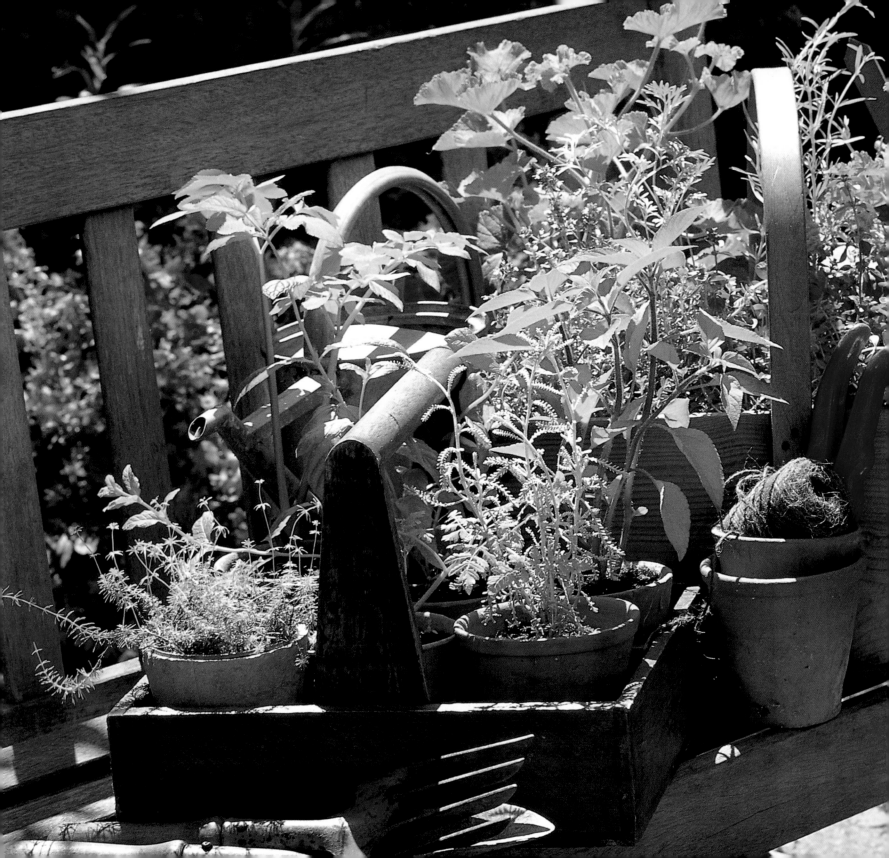

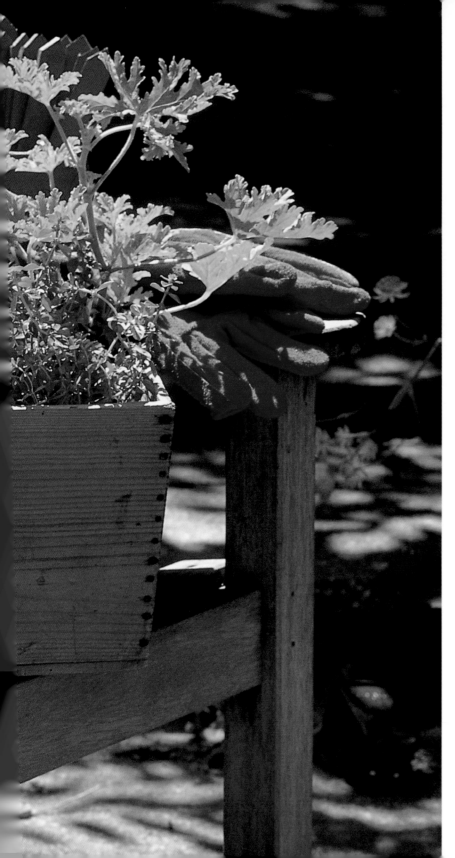

CHAPTER ONE

GROWING HERBS

"Anything green that grew out of the mould
Was an excellent herb to our fathers of old."
RUDYARD KIPLING

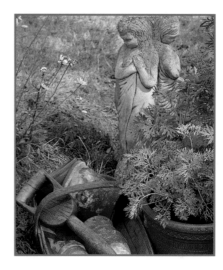

One of the best ways of ensuring that you have the raw materials to hand for making simple home remedies is to grow your own herbs: this way you can be sure they have not been sprayed with chemicals or unhygienically harvested or stored.

This chapter begins with tips on starting a herb garden and includes plenty of ideas for growing herbs in pots. There is also advice on how to propagate and get your plants going in the first place.

ABOVE: Wormwood, Artemisia absinthum, *has insect-repellent properties. Grow it in a pot or among other herbs in the garden to deter pests.*

LEFT: Growing your own plants ensures a ready source of ingredients for herbal remedies.

PLANTING A HERB GARDEN

You don't need very much space to grow herbs. A small border or bed, or even a collection of containers, will provide an adequate supply of plants for household needs. If you do have the room, of course, a full-scale herb garden makes a rewarding and decorative feature as well as having a practical purpose.

Soil

On the whole, herbs are undemanding and easy to grow. A free-draining, lightish soil will suit the majority. They are essentially wild plants, and the one thing they do not require is the rich, highly cultivated soil necessary for successful vegetable crops and garden flowers.

Many of the most useful herbs, such as sage, thyme, rosemary and lavender, are from the Mediterranean region and will not stand heavy clay soils or water-logged conditions. Those species found on clay soils in the wild, such as comfrey or sweet cicely – which favours moist loam – are vigorous and adaptable enough to grow anywhere.

Even naturally moisture-loving plants, such as angelica, lemon balm and valerian, will grow happily in a light soil, though not in conditions of total drought. The same goes for most of the mints: their growth will not be strong in a light, sandy soil, but in view of their thuggish reputation you may consider this an advantage.

RIGHT: A formal framework of rectangular beds and gravel paths keeps herbs under control and makes cultivation and picking easier.

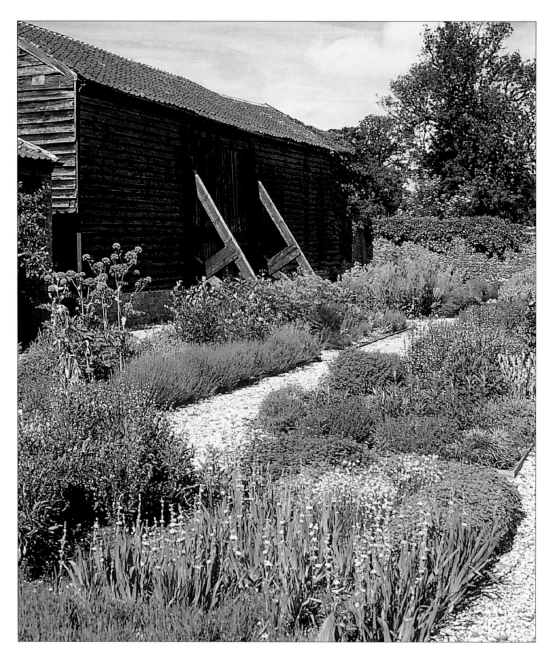

10

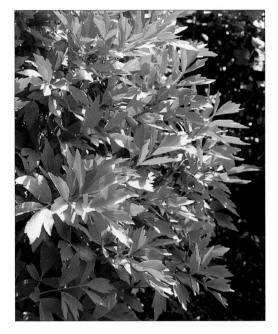

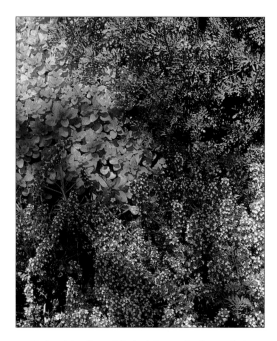

LEFT: Lovage grows prolifically – cut it back ruthlessly to prevent it overpowering its neighbours.

RIGHT (CLOCKWISE FROM FRONT): Thyme, golden marjoram and rue.

Site

A sunny, sheltered position protected from biting winter winds will suit the plants best. Silvery plants, thymes, lavender and rosemary will not withstand harsh winters. Some plants, such as lemon verbena and bay, are not totally hardy and will need winter protection. The useful *Aloe vera* is an exotic which tolerates no frost at all and must be treated as a houseplant in colder regions.

Design

A formal, symmetrical layout of small beds, dissected by gravel or paved paths, provides a framework for the lax, untidy growth of many herbs. It also makes tending and harvesting the plants easier. Beds can be edged with clipped dwarf hedges, tiles or simple boarding. A

RIGHT: A bay tree in a pot makes a focal point in the herb garden.

single species in each bed can look most attractive and was the favoured design for the apothecaries' gardens of medieval times.

In complete contrast, an informal cottage-garden style provides plenty of scope for imaginative, exuberant planting. It also requires a little less maintenance than the more formal designs.

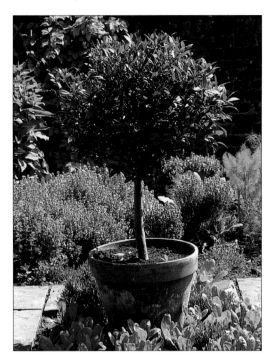

Raised beds, with brick or timber edging, make easy-to-control, self-contained herb gardens. They are ideal if you are gardening on heavy clay since they can be filled with the appropriate soil over a layer of rubble.

Maintenance

Many herbs are prolific growers. Harvesting them for use in home-made preparations helps to keep them under control, but do not be afraid to cut them back ruthlessly from time to time and root out those that are overpowering their neighbours.

Weeding is important to prevent competition for moisture and nutrients. A light mulch of good, home-made garden compost or manure, applied in spring or autumn, can help to keep the herbs in good heart.

Most herbs will withstand dry summers, but coriander, parsley and chervil are apt to bolt if it is too dry, and may need watering.

SOWING SEEDS

Many herbs are easy to grow from seed, so this is a good way to stock your garden inexpensively. Spring is generally the best time for sowing. There is no virtue in starting too early when temperatures and light levels are low; seeds sown slightly later will produce stronger plants. Chervil and coriander can be sown in the autumn to give them a good start.

Seeds can be sown outdoors in spring but will be at the mercy of the weather and hungry birds. Sowing in seed trays is a surer way to success – especially for parsley, which needs heat to germinate.

YOU WILL NEED
cellular seed tray
soilless seed and potting compost (growing medium)
watering can
herb seeds
sieve
polythene (plastic) dome or plastic bag
label
7.5cm/3in pots

—GERMINATION—
Most plants from temperate areas will germinate at 10–13°C/50–55°F. Plants from warmer regions, including basil, germinate best at about 15°C/60°F. Parsley needs a higher temperature, 18–21°C/65–70°F and rosemary 27–32°C/80–90°F.

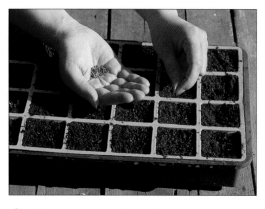

1 Fill a seed tray with soilless compost (growing medium). A tray divided into cells makes it easier to sow thinly and to pot up seedlings. Water first, then scatter two or three seeds in each compartment.

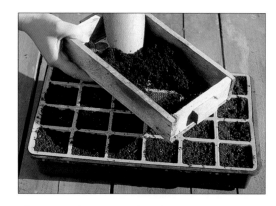

2 Cover the tray with a thin layer of sieved compost. Never bury seeds too deeply, especially small ones such as parsley. Water again very lightly and don't forget to label the tray (seedlings all look very similar when they have just germinated).

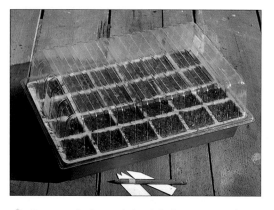

3 Put a polythene (plastic) dome over the tray, or enclose it in a plastic bag, to retain moisture. Put the tray on a windowsill or in the greenhouse and cover with black polythene until the seedlings begin to show.

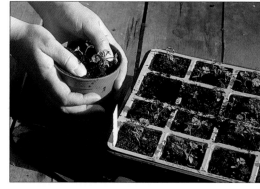

4 When the seedlings come through, remove the cover and put the tray in a light place out of direct sunlight. Keep moist, but never waterlogged. As soon as the seedlings are large enough to handle, pot them up individually in 7.5cm/3in pots filled with fresh potting compost.

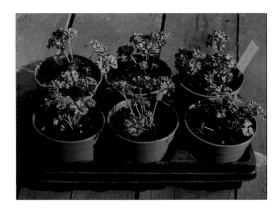

5 Once the plants have put on some strong growth, they can be potted on into larger containers, or planted out in the garden.

RIGHT: Growing your own herbs from seed is an easy and inexpensive way to stock your garden.

—HERBS TO GROW FROM SEED—
ANNUALS
basil, borage, chervil, coriander, dill, nasturtium, pot marigold, summer savory

BIENNIALS
angelica, clary sage, parsley (best treated as an annual, sowing seed every spring)

PERENNIALS
fennel, feverfew, horehound (slow to germinate), hyssop (but to perpetuate a particular colour, take cuttings), lovage, winter savory

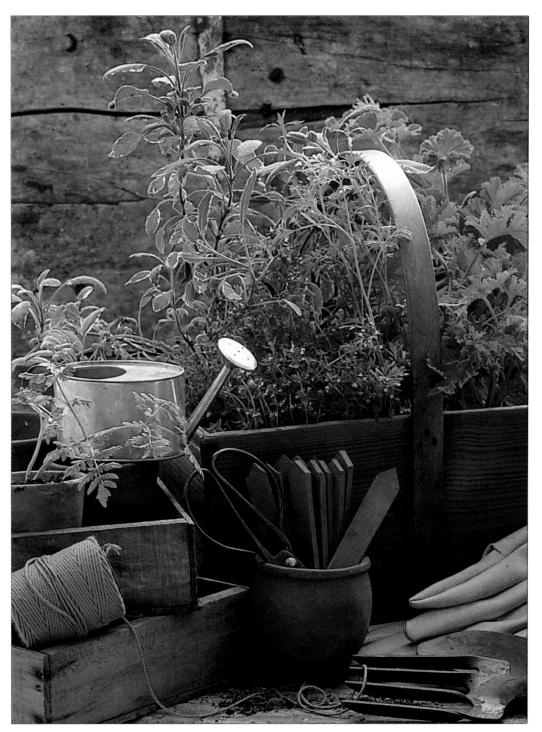

DIVIDING PLANTS

Division is the best way to increase herbs with fibrous roots, such as chives and marjoram, and also those with fleshy tap-roots, including lovage and comfrey. Chives need dividing every few years for vigorous growth.

YOU WILL NEED
garden fork
chives
7.5cm/3in pots
all-purpose compost (growing medium)
secateurs (pruners) or scissors

BELOW: *Chive flowers*

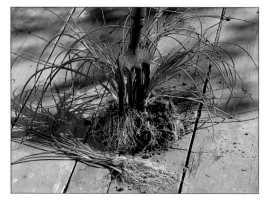

1 Dig up a clump of chives and divide it into several new pieces, pulling it apart with the aid of a small fork.

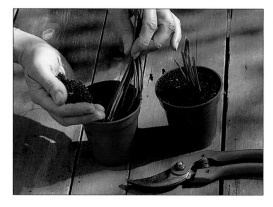

2 Firm each new piece into a pot filled with all-purpose compost (growing medium). Cut off some of the top-growth and water.

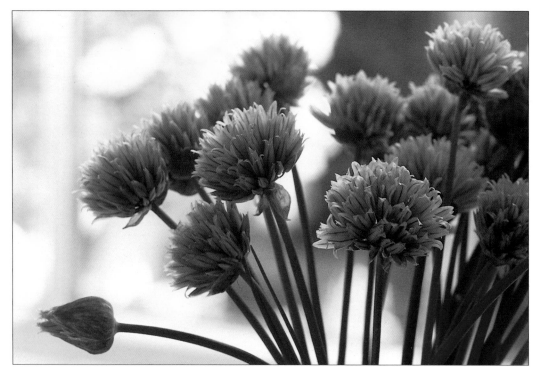

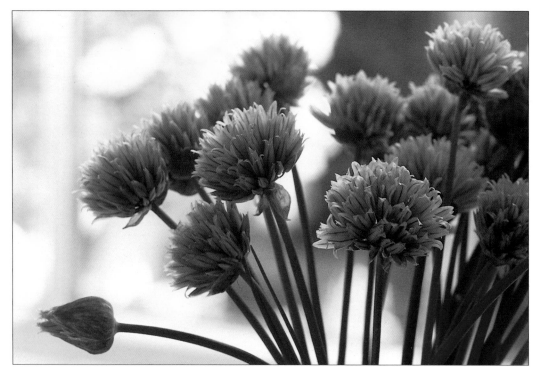

3 The new plants will soon grow strongly to provide plenty of fresh leaf.

—HERBS TO GROW FROM ROOT
DIVISION OR OFF-SETS—
chamomile, chives, comfrey, horseradish,
houseleek, lovage, marjoram, mint,
soapwort, tarragon

ROOT CUTTINGS

Herbs with creeping root systems such as mint, tarragon, soapwort and bugle, are easy to propagate by cutting their roots into separate pieces to form new plants. Invasive plants such as mint are best grown in separate containers for maximum convenience and to prevent them spreading and taking over the garden. Mint has so many uses, from making teas for the relief of indigestion or colds to scenting the bath water, that it is always useful to have a good supply.

YOU WILL NEED
garden fork
mint
secateurs (pruners) or scissors
seed tray
all-purpose compost (growing medium)
watering can
7.5cm/3in pots (optional)

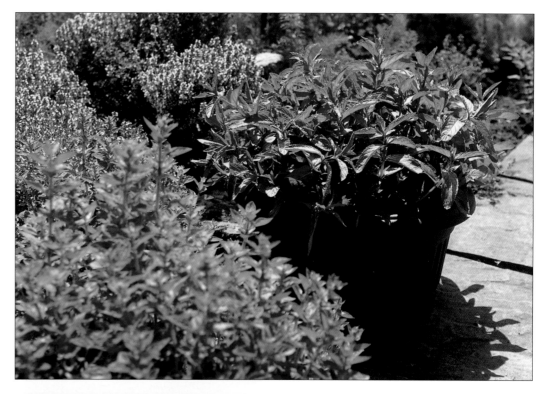

ABOVE: Container-grown mint needs to be split up and re-potted every year as the roots become very congested. It can also be grown in a bucket with no base buried in the soil.

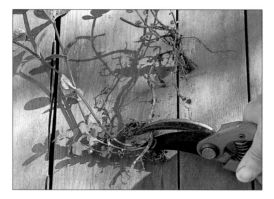

1 Lift a root of mint and cut it into 4cm 1½in pieces at each joint where there is a developing shoot.

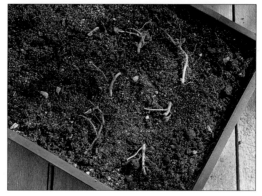

2 Fill a seed tray with all-purpose compost (growing medium). Lay the pieces of root on the surface, press them in lightly and cover with a further layer of compost. Water well and leave in a shady place indoors or out. There is no need to cover the tray or enclose it in polythene, but do keep it moist.

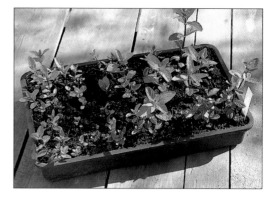

3 Once there are plenty of leaves showing, divide the new plants and grow them on in bigger pots or in the open ground.

15

STEM CUTTINGS

Some plants are best propagated from cuttings. This is either because they do not set seed, or because they produce seedlings that are not true to the parent plant. Shrubby herbs such as southernwood, thyme, rosemary and lavender should be propagated from cuttings.

YOU WILL NEED
plants
sharp knife or secateurs (pruners)
15cm/6in pot
cuttings compost (growing medium)
hormone rooting powder
dibber (dibble) pencil or stick
polythene (plastic) dome or plastic bag

—*PROPAGATING SAGE*—
Sages are also usually propagated from cuttings, but they vary as to the ease of the process. Pineapple sage *(Salvia rutilans)* strikes very easily from softwood cuttings taken throughout the growing season. Purple and golden sage cuttings take less readily and it is easier to "layer" these plants. Simply peg an outer stem down into the soil until new roots are formed at the junction (this takes several months). Don't forget to water the "layer" in dry spells. The purple and golden varieties do not set seed, but common sage *(Salvia officinalis)* is easy to grow by this method.

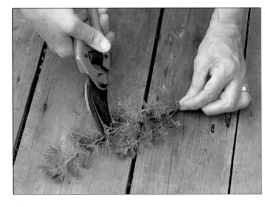

1 Choose a stem from the new growth of the plant (in this case, southernwood). Cut it into sections just below each leaf joint. Remove all but the top two or three leaves from each cutting.

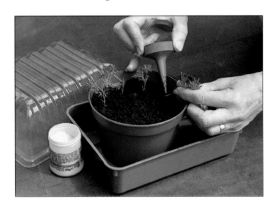

2 Fill a pot with cuttings compost (growing medium), tapping it down to exclude air. Dip the cuttings into hormone rooting powder, and firm them into the compost around the edge of the pot. Cover with a polythene (plastic) dome or plastic bag and place out of direct sunlight until rooted.

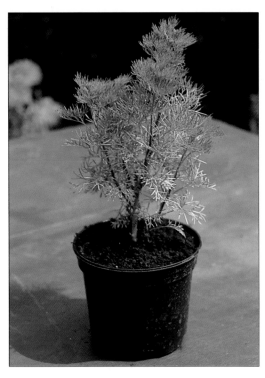

3 When a good root system has developed and the cuttings have put on plenty of new growth (this will take 2–3 weeks) they can be planted out or potted up into larger pots. Southernwood is likely to become straggly after 4–5 years, but new plants strike easily.

HERBS TO GROW FROM CUTTINGS
bay (slow), cotton lavender, elder, hyssop, lavender, pineapple sage, pinks, rosemary, scented-leaf pelargoniums, southernwood, thyme, wormwood

OFF-SETS

Some plants, such as chamomile and house-leek, spread by sending out runners. It's a simple matter to increase your stock by potting up the off-sets (offshoots).

YOU WILL NEED
garden fork
plants
secateurs (pruners)
7.5cm/3in pots
gritty compost (growing medium)
horticultural sand or grit
watering can

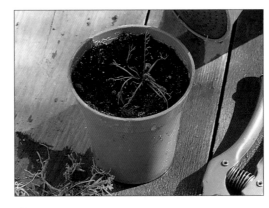

2 Press each new plantlet into a pot of compost (growing medium). Water and leave in a shady place until new roots develop.

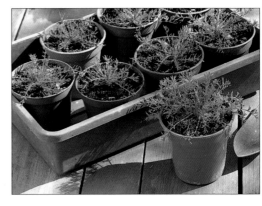

3 The cuttings will grow into bushy plants in 2–3 weeks, when they can be potted on into larger pots or planted out in the garden.

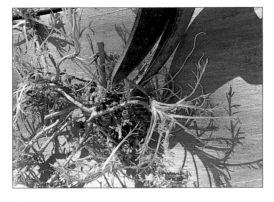

1 Lift a chamomile plant and separate the satellite off-sets (offshoots).

RIGHT: Houseleek (Sempervivum tectorum) *is a useful plant for soothing skin irritations.*

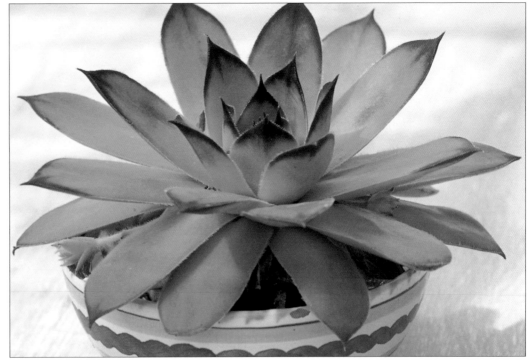

GROWING IN CONTAINERS

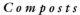

Most of the herbs you will need can be grown in containers. Some, such as bay, sage, thyme and lemon verbena, can be kept in the same pot for several seasons. Others, such as mints, will need splitting up every year as their roots become entangled. Annuals, of course, are started afresh each spring.

Container Size

When planting several species of herbs together, make sure you choose a container large enough to give the roots room to spread out. But remember that this is usually a short-term exercise; close, mixed plantings need re-doing annually. If you grow a single variety in a large pot, the plants can stay put longer and you will get plenty of leaf to cut.

Drainage

Good drainage is one of the keys to success. Make sure there are holes in the base of the pot. Put in a layer of crocks (broken terracotta pots), then cover with a layer of sand or grit before filling with potting compost (soil mix).

Composts

It's important to use the right mix of compost in a container. Potting composts (soil mix) come in two main types: the John Innes formulae, based on sterilized loam, and the soilless composts (growing medium) based on peat or peat substitutes such as coir. Never use garden soil: it will not provide enough nutrients and may harbour weeds, pests and diseases.

Soilless composts (growing mediums) are lighter and easier to handle, but they do not retain nutrients as long as the loam-based (soil mix) ones. They provide a moister environment for the plant but, if left unwatered, they also dry out more quickly, shrink from the side of the pot and are extremely difficult to re-moisten.

Most herbs flourish in a free-draining compost (soil mix) and, as a general rule, a 3:1 mixture of soilless and loam-based composts provides the best results. A few handfuls of fine grit added to the mix will open the texture and improve drainage. This is especially important for shrubby herbs and scented pelargoniums.

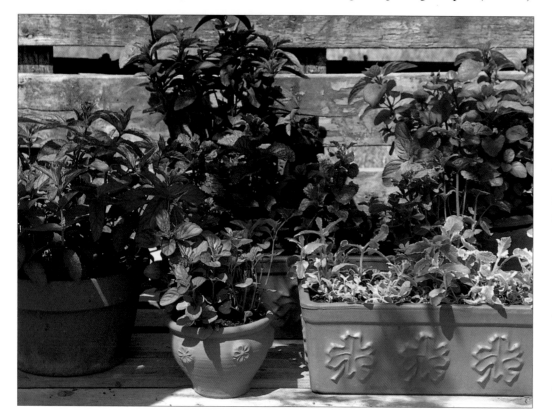

LEFT (CLOCKWISE FROM FRONT): Eau-de-Cologne mint (ideal for revitalizing baths), spearmint (best for cooking), peppermint, eau-de-Cologne mint, variegated applemint (for baths and pot-pourri). (CENTRE): Moroccan mint (for tea).

Feeding

Both the loam-based and soilless composts are available containing nutrients in a range of proportions. "Seed and cuttings" compost (soil mix) contains the least, and "potting" compost the most, with "all-purpose" somewhere in between. Use either of the last two for container-grown plants. Extra fertilizer must be added after 4 weeks, with subsequent weekly feeds throughout the growing season. An organic plant food based on seaweed extract is preferable but, to save time, slow-release fertilizer added at the time of potting-up can also be used.

Watering

Pot-grown plants need frequent watering during the growing season. As a general rule, it is better to let them almost dry out and then give them a good soaking than to keep dribbling in small amounts of water. Some of the culinary herbs, especially basil and coriander, do better if kept more consistently moist. Water-retaining gel mixed into the compost at the time of planting makes watering less of a chore. During the winter months perennials kept in pots should be given the minimum amount of water possible.

RIGHT: Lemon verbena (LEFT) and tricolour sage (RIGHT) can be left in the same container for several years, but mixed plantings have a shorter life and annuals, like these colourful nasturtiums (FRONT), only last for one season.

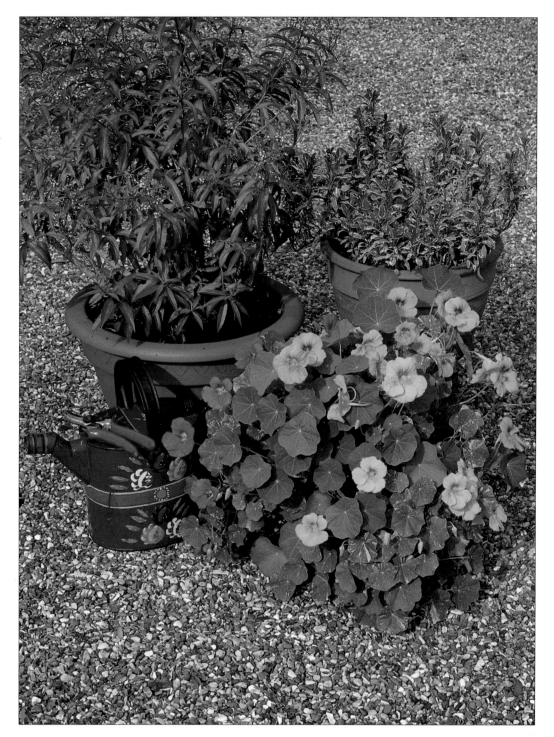

HARVESTING AND STORING HERBS

Fresh herbs can be picked at any time during the growing season, whenever you need them. Obviously it makes sense to let young plants develop before harvesting them too much. Evergreens can also be picked to use fresh during the winter, but only very sparingly, as they will not be putting on new growth; nor will they have the same therapeutic properties while dormant as in the summer when the essential oil content is at its height. Herbs which die off or die back at the end of the growing season need to be harvested when at their best, then dried and stored for later use.

Gathering

When harvesting for drying, pick flowers at their peak before they start to go over. Herbs required for their leaves should be picked before flowering. Snipping off flower-buds

BELOW: Lovage leaves, spread out on paper, have been dried in a warm airing-cupboard to keep a good colour.

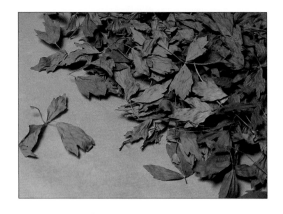

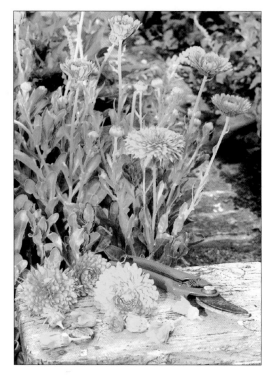

before they can form encourages a longer period of leafy growth. Shrubby and non-flowering herbs can be harvested at any time throughout the growing season.

Never cut herbs or flowers for drying on a wet day. The optimum time – though this is less important – is in the morning after the dew has evaporated but before the sun has released too much of the essential oil.

Drying

The secret of drying herbs successfully is to remove the moisture without sacrificing too much of the essential oil content. This is

achieved by drying at the correct temperature. A boiler room or airing-cupboard is an ideal place. Failing that, a warm, airy room is a good compromise, or even a garden shed, provided it is completely dry. If possible, avoid drying herbs or flowers in direct sunlight.

LEFT: Pot marigold flowers are picked for drying before they have a chance to go over. Plants for drying should be in the best possible condition.

BELOW: A small lavender bundle drying.

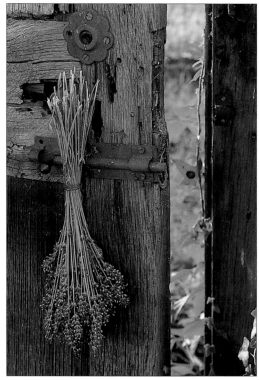

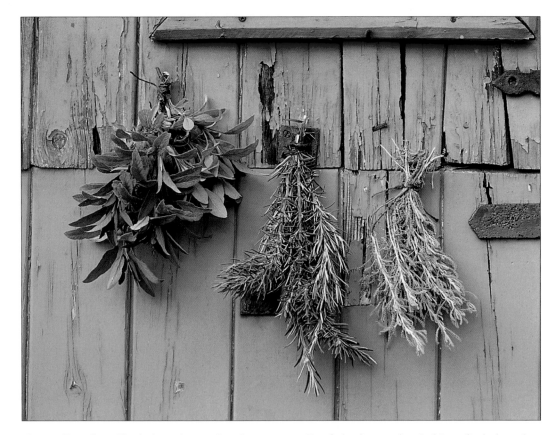

ABOVE: Bunches of herbs hanging to dry. (FROM LEFT) Purple sage, rosemary and cotton lavender.

BELOW: Storing dried lovage for culinary use.

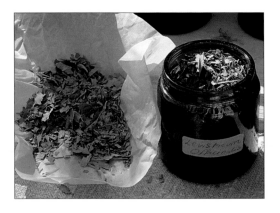

Leafy herbs can be tied into little bunches and hung up, or they can be spread out in orange-boxes set on top of each other. Tie lavender stems in bunches to dry – it's a good idea to suspend them with the heads inside brown paper bags to exclude dust and catch any petals that drop. Spread flowers on tissue or newspaper, leaving them whole or twisting the petals off the heads. Leave herbs and flowers until papery dry to the touch. This can take up to a week.

Storing

Rub leafy herbs off their stems as soon as they are dry. The job is easier if you wear light cotton gloves.

Dried herbs deteriorate quickly if left out in the light and air. Keep them in a cool, dark place. Dark glass or pottery jars make the best containers. Herbs also keep well in sealed brown paper bags. This is particularly useful for heads of lavender.

Cellophane bags are fine for keeping herbs for short periods but don't use polythene (plastic) bags or containers as they draw out residual moisture in the dried material. Dried herbs should not be exposed to any dampness. If left in unsealed containers, they will take in moisture from the surrounding air.

Although many dried herbs retain an aromatic scent for several years, for culinary and medicinal purposes it is best to replace stocks every year since their potency declines with age. Drying your own herbs allows you to know exactly how old your stock is.

BELOW: Pot marigolds, dried in the summer when they are plentiful, can be made into healing salves and ointments.

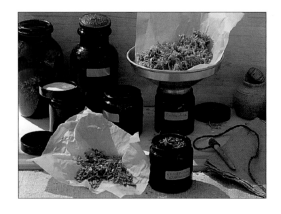

AN INDOOR HERB GARDEN

It is best to think of growing herbs indoors as a temporary measure, for convenience when cooking. They need light and air to flourish and are happier outside. A good way to see that they thrive is to alternate pots of culinary herbs on the windowsill with another set left standing outside, where they will have time to recover from constant cutting. Keep the different herbs in individual 17cm/6½in pots, and group them together in a single container. Standing the pots on gravel keeps them cool and helps to retain moisture. The plants grow better in close proximity to one another because transpiration from the massed leaves increases the overall humidity slightly.

YOU WILL NEED
window box or other large container
drill, if necessary
gravel or horticultural grit
trowel
watering can
herbs in pots
drip tray

PLANTS
SPRING AND SUMMER: *basil, chervil, chives, coriander, dill, mint, parsley, tarragon*
AUTUMN AND WINTER: *bay, marjoram, rosemary, sage, thyme, winter savory*

RIGHT: *A second set of individually potted herbs, kept outside, can be alternated with those in an indoor container.*

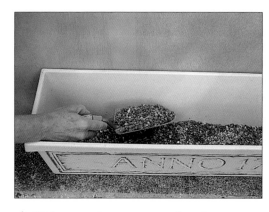

1 Make sure the outer container has drainage holes drilled in the base and, if not, use a drill to make some. Put a shallow layer of gravel or horticultural grit into the container so that the top of each pot will be just below the rim of the container.

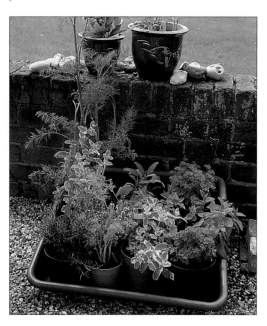

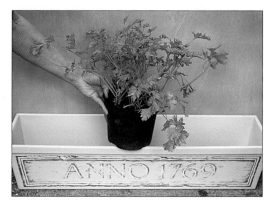

2 Water each pot well, then stand it on the gravel layer.

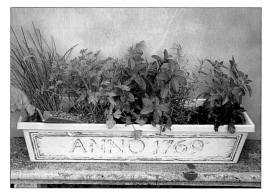

3 When all the pots are in place, fill around the tops with extra gravel. New pots can be substituted at any time. Lift out the one you wish to change and bed the new one into the gravel in its place.

OPPOSITE (LEFT TO RIGHT): *Chives, flat-leafed parsley, mint, French tarragon, green and purple basil. Grouping individual pots in a container is a practical way to grow herbs.*

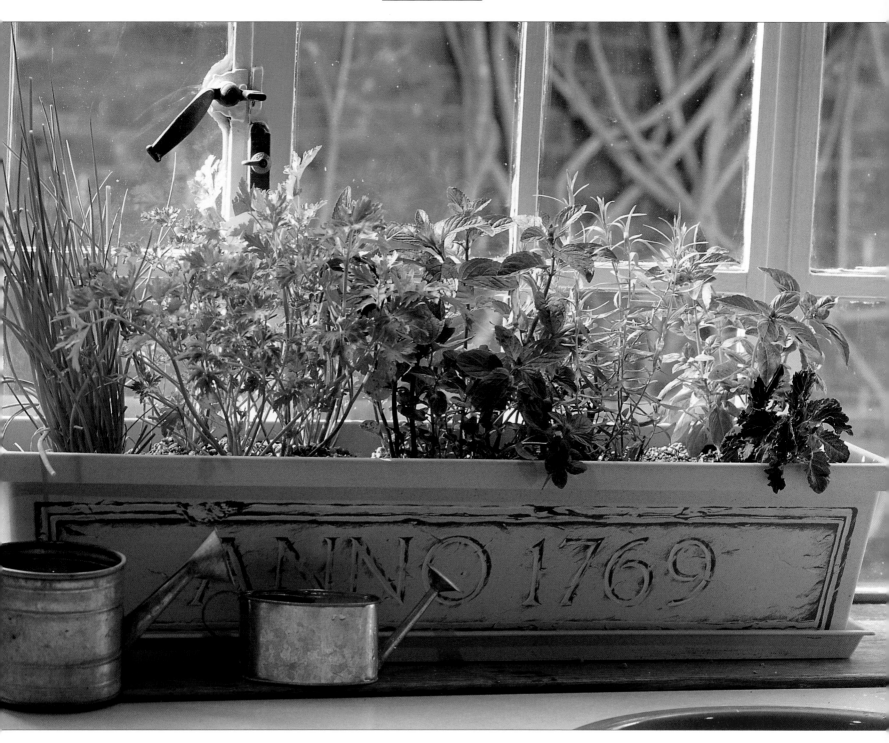

A Thyme Pot for Youthful Vigour

Thyme's antiseptic properties make it a number one choice for treating sore throats, coughs and colds. The essential oil contains a high level of antioxidants and recent research has established a link between taking thyme essential oil and slowing down the ageing process.

Fortunately, thyme is easy to grow in pots so you can always have a ready supply. It adapts well to living in a planter with holes in the sides, which makes a colourful and attractive patio or garden feature.

You will need
slow-release fertilizer
water-retaining gel
soilless compost (growing medium)
loam-based compost (soil mix)
trowel
terracotta pot with planting pockets
crocks (broken terracotta pots)
watering can
shallow container

Plants
MEDICINAL USE: *common thyme (*Thymus vulgaris), *wild or creeping thyme*
(T. serpyllum, T. serpyllum *var*. albus, T. serpyllum *'Annie Hall')*
CULINARY USE: *lemon thyme* (T. x citriodorus), *golden thyme* (T. x citriodorus *'Archer's Gold')*

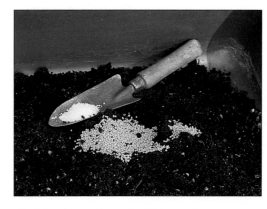

1 Mix slow-release fertilizer and water-retaining gel, following the manufacturer's instructions, into a potting medium made up of equal parts of soilless (growing medium) and loam-based composts (soil mix).

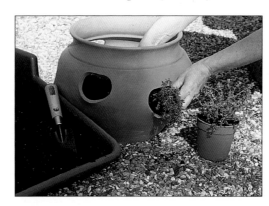

2 Choose a planter with generously sized pockets so that the plants are not squashed. Put a layer of crocks (broken terracotta pots) in the bottom and fill to the first hole with the prepared potting medium. Tap a thyme plant out of its pot and feed it through the hole, working from the inside out.

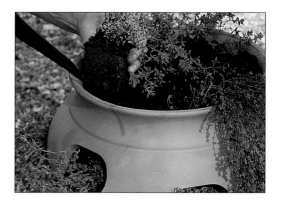

3 Cover the roots with more compost and firm it down before adding a further layer. Put in more plants until all the holes are filled. Plant the top with one or more good, bushy specimens and water in thoroughly.

— Maintenance —
Water regularly, but allow the compost almost to dry out between waterings. For tall thyme planters, water from beneath as well as on top. The same planting should last from year to year if you keep the pot in a sheltered place during the winter. Trim any shaggy growth in the spring and feed with a liquid fertilizer.

OPPOSITE: *The top is planted with* T. vulgaris *(white flower),* 'Silver Posie' *(variegated) and* T. serpyllum *(mauve flower), with more* T. vulgaris *in the pocket on the left and* 'Archer's Gold' *on the right.*

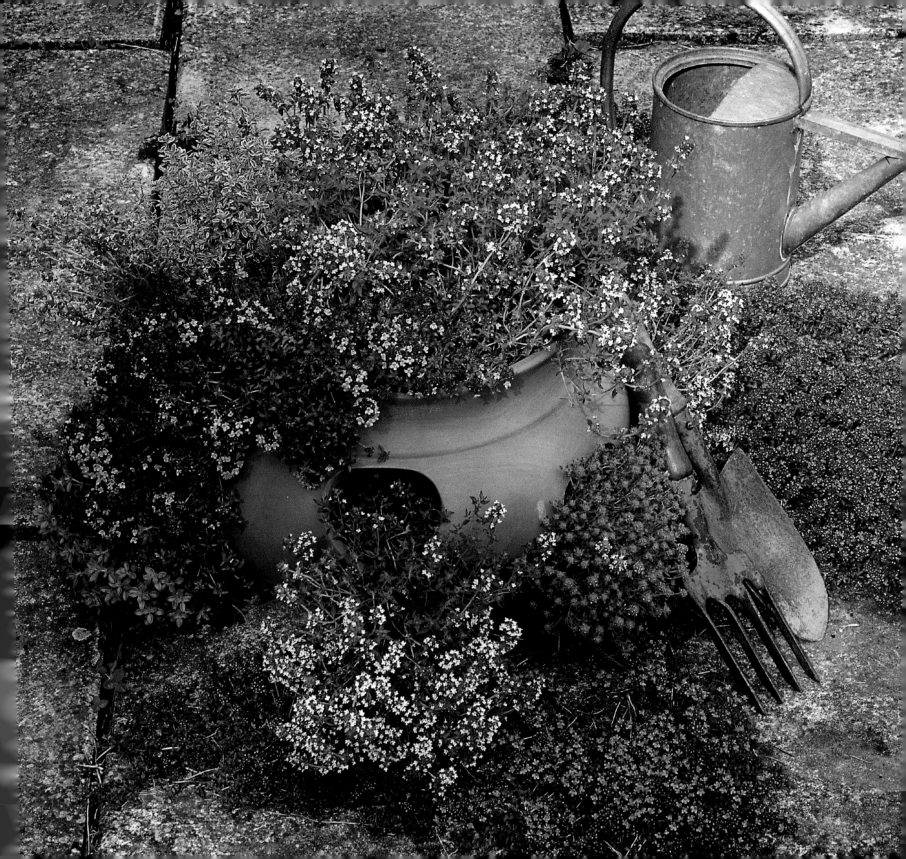

A FRAGRANT BASKET FOR RELAXATION

When the pace of life becomes too much, a short relaxation break sitting somewhere peaceful surrounded by the scent of herbs and flowers helps to restore calm. A hanging basket is ideal for providing scent at nose level. Hang it in a rose garden, suspended near a comfortable seat with a tub of lemon verbena or lavender nearby, to create a cocoon of relaxing fragrance.

YOU WILL NEED
35cm/14in diameter hanging basket
bucket
fibre basket liner or moss
hanging-basket compost (growing medium)
watering can

PLANTS
bugle (Ajuga reptans *'Atropurpurea'*,
A. reptans *'Tricolor'*)
creeping pennyroyal (Mentha pulegium)
creeping thyme (T. serpyllum)
Cheddar pink (Dianthus gratianopolitanus)
maiden pink (Dianthus deltoides)
scented-leaf pelargoniums (P. *'Sweet Mimosa'*,
P. *'Fragrans Variegatum'*, P. *'Graveolens'*, or
P. *tomentosum*)
Verbena (V. *'Sissinghurst'*)

— MAINTENANCE —
The basket will need watering every day.
In very hot, dry weather you may need
to water twice a day.

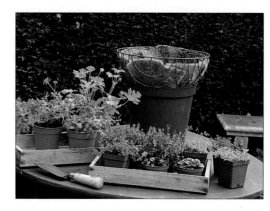

1 Stand the basket on a bucket to give it stability while you work. Put in a liner of fibre or moss.

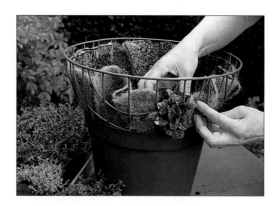

2 Half-fill with hanging-basket compost (growing medium) and ease the first plant (this is the bugle, *Ajuga reptans 'Atropurpurea'*) through the side. Plant the sides with creeping pennyroyal, creeping thyme and small pinks, topping up with more compost as you go. If planting gaps seem tight, wrap the foliage in a cone of newspaper before pushing it through.

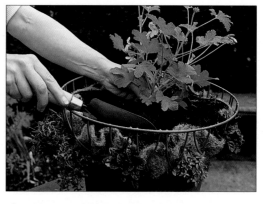

3 Put a scented-leaf pelargonium (P. 'Sweet Mimosa') in the top at the centre, filling around it with more compost.

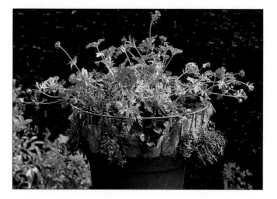

4 Finish the planting with three *Verbena* 'Sissinghurst', around the rim of the basket, firming the plants into place. Water well and leave to settle in a greenhouse or sheltered place for two or three days. Hang the basket in its final position after any risk of frost.

OPPOSITE: *A basket of fragrant plants provides scent at head height.*

26

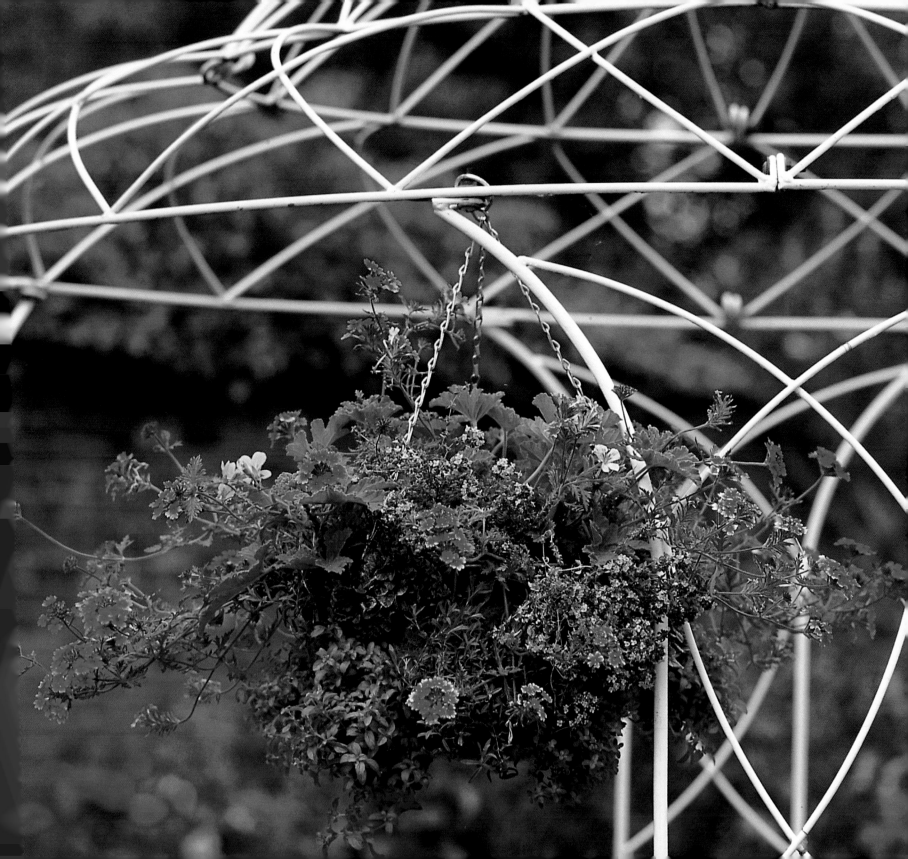

A TROUGH FOR WARDING OFF WINTER COLDS

A collection of herbs for use in teas and other cold remedies is useful at any time of the year. Most of them, including thyme, sage, horehound and, to a lesser extent, hyssop, keep their leaves through the winter when they can still be picked in small quantities, but they do not have the same potency while dormant, so harvest them while they are growing vigorously and dry them for later use.

YOU WILL NEED
trough
crocks (broken terracotta pots)
gravel or horticultural grit
potting compost (soil mix)
watering can

PLANTS
black peppermint (Mentha *x* piperita)
hyssop (Hyssopus officinalis)
horehound (Marrubium vulgare)
sage (Salvia officinalis)
purple sage (S. officinalis purpurea)
golden sage (S. officinalis 'Icterina')
thymes (Thymus vulgaris, T. *x* citriodorus 'Aureus', T. vulgaris 'Silver Posie', T. serpyllum, T. richardii *ssp*. nitidus 'Peter Davis')

— MAINTENANCE —
Do not let the trough dry out and feed every 2–3 weeks with a liquid fertilizer during the growing season. Replant annually, using fresh compost.

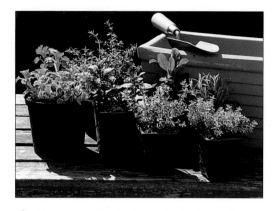

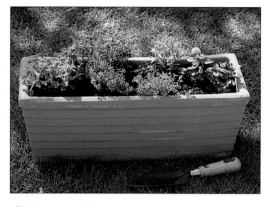

1 Make sure the drainage holes in the bottom of the container are open. Put in a layer of crocks (broken terracotta pots), topped with a layer of gravel or horticultural grit and fill with a good quality potting compost (soil mix). Leave plenty of room for the plants.

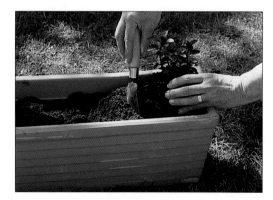

2 Position the plants while they are still in their pots, then tap them out and plant, firming around each one with extra compost. Put the tallest plants (horehound, hyssop, sage and peppermint) at the back and the thymes at the front.

3 Top up with extra compost as necessary and water the plants in well. It is best to replant a mixed container like this anually to prevent the plants becoming overgrown.

OPPOSITE: Two troughs planted with herbs for cold remedies provide extra plants for cutting and make an attractive garden feature.

BELOW (CLOCKWISE FROM FRONT): 'Peter Davis', 'Silver Posie', golden thyme, horehound, hyssop and black peppermint.

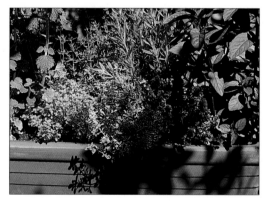

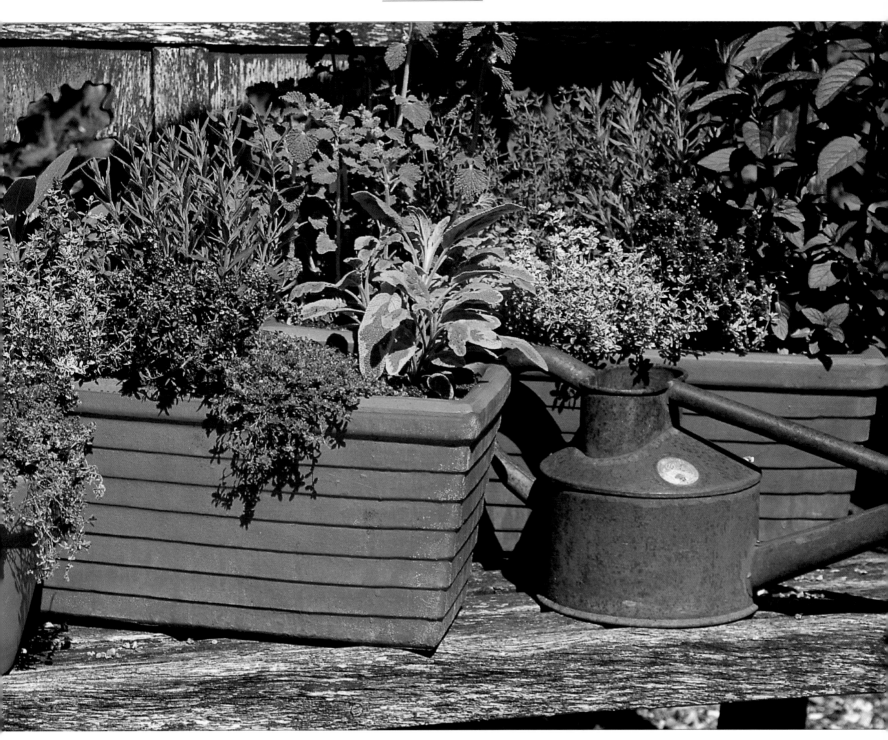

A TUB FOR HEADACHE REMEDIES

Many herbs are helpful in relieving headaches brought on by tension and anxiety. The plants can be used fresh, or dried, and made into teas or compresses. Feverfew's ability to reduce migraine attacks has been well documented; the classic way to take it is to eat two or three leaves daily in a brown bread sandwich to disguise the bitter taste.

A half-barrel makes a practical container as it gives the plants plenty of room to grow. It is extremely heavy and impossible to move once filled, so site it where you want it to stay.

YOU WILL NEED
half-barrel
bricks
heavy-duty black polythene (plastic)
staples
hammer
knife
crocks (broken terracotta pots)
horticultural grit
soilless compost (growing medium)
sharp sand
watering can

PLANTS
feverfew (Tanacetum parthenium)
lavender (Lavandula *'Hidcote'*, L. stoechas)
marjoram (Origanum vulgare *'Variegatum'*)
rosemary (Rosmarinus officinalis), *prostrate
and upright forms*
St John's wort (Hypericum perforatum)

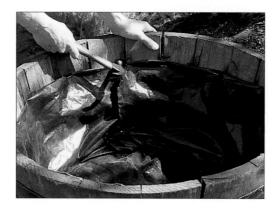

1 Rest the tub on a few bricks to raise it off the ground. Insert the plastic liner and staple it to the side. Make some drainage holes in the base. Put in a layer of crocks (broken terracotta pots), topped with grit. Add soilless compost (growing medium), mixed with sand, to come a third of the way up the tub.

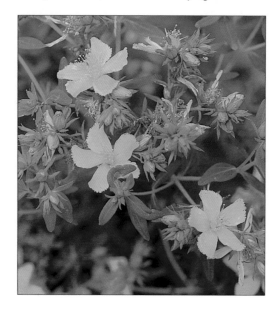

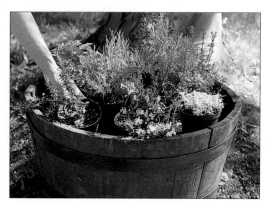

2 Fill almost to the top with a gritty, open-textured potting compost (growing medium). Arrange the herbs, still in their pots, to decide on their final positions in the tub. They can be planted fairly close together, but be sure to leave them plenty of growing room. Plant and water in well.

LEFT: St John's wort (Hypericum perforatum).

OPPOSITE: In a tub this size, the plants can be left for several years without disturbance. Keep them well trimmed, replace the top layer of compost annually and feed regularly in the summer months.

—CAUTION—
Eating too many feverfew leaves over a prolonged period may cause mouth ulcers. Anyone suffering from severe or frequent headaches should consult a medical practitioner.

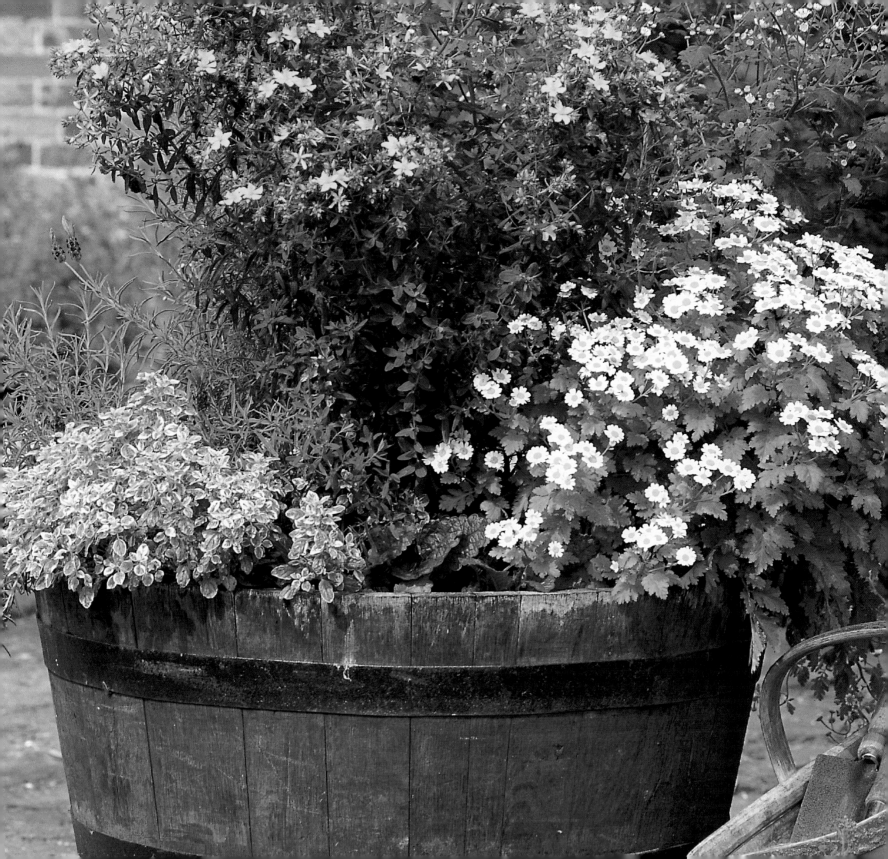

A POTTED TEA GARDEN

If a plant is to be picked frequently to make herbal tea and a good supply of leaves is required for drying, it pays to grow it in its own pot rather than in a mixed tub, where development is often curtailed. For fully grown plants, use a container with a minimum diameter of 23cm/9in, though larger plants will do better in a 30cm/12in pot.

Buy lemon verbena and bergamot plants and pot up into larger containers. You can start peppermint and chamomile from cuttings if you have access to garden plants. Dill, borage and caraway are easy to grow from seed.

Rosemary, sage and thyme could also be included for a more comprehensive selection. Group the pots for ease of access – the plants also benefit from growing near each other.

PLANTS
bergamot (Monarda didyma)
borage (Borago officinalis)
caraway (Carum carvi)
chamomile (Chamaemelum nobile)
dill (Anethum graveolens)
lemon verbena (Aloysia triphylla)
peppermint (Mentha *x* piperita)

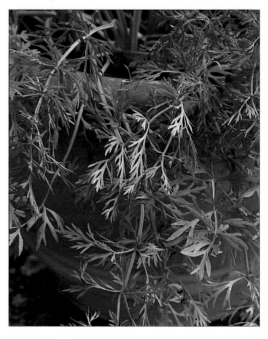

ABOVE: *Collect the seeds from a caraway plant to make a digestive tea.*

LEFT: *A group of containers provides the raw materials for herbal teas.*

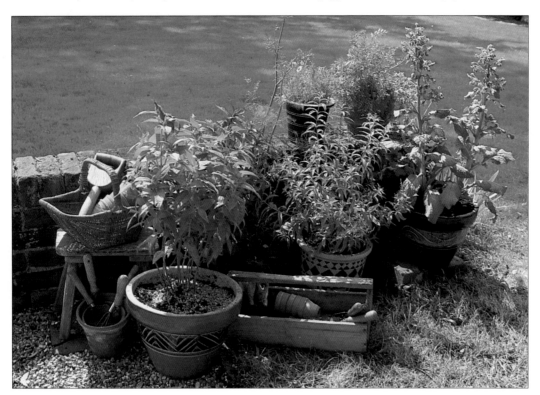

— MAINTENANCE —
Peppermint should be re-potted every year. Chamomile off-sets (offshoots) can be replanted when the foliage becomes too crowded. Dill and borage are annuals and will need to be started fresh each year, though caraway, being a biennial, will last for two. You can keep lemon verbena in the same pot for several years.

An Insect-repellent Collection

Many garden herbs have insect-repellent properties. They can be dried to put into sachets for your wardrobe or linen cupboard and made into a variety of preparations and lotions. They can also be grown among other garden plants as deterrents to insect pests – chives and garlic are especially effective for this. For a ready source of material for insect-repellent recipes, keep a collection of suitable herbs in containers. Plant them in individual pots or put two or three different plants together in one pot.

BELOW: Pennyroyal is disliked by ants – keep a pot on the patio.

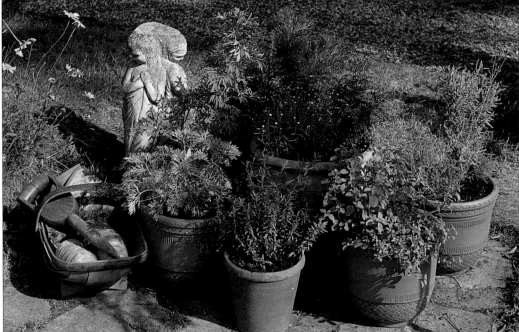

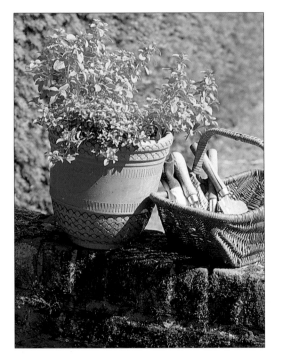

Pennyroyal is disliked by ants, so keep a pot where they are prevalent. Southernwood, cotton lavender, rue and hyssop can be dried for inclusion in sachets and wormwood makes an effective anti-insect lotion.

PLANTS
cotton lavender (Santolina pinnata, *'Edward Bowles'* Santolina virens)
hyssop (Hyssopus officinalis)
pennyroyal (Mentha pulegium) *creeping and upright forms*
rue (Ruta graveolens *'Jackman's Blue'*)
southernwood (Artemisia abrotanum)
wormwood (Artemisia absinthum)

ABOVE: A collection of insect-repellent herbs.

— *MAINTENANCE* —
Trim straggly growth and re-pot as they outgrow their containers. Pennyroyal is hardy, but most of the others which have silvery foliage will need winter protection.

— *CAUTION* —
Rue is an irritant plant which can cause severe blisters. Do not let it brush the skin, and only handle wearing gloves.

A Container for Bites and Bruises

A stone trough or basin makes a good container for plants used to make salves and ointments to counteract the effects of bites and bruises. It is best to grow the tall form of comfrey, *Symphytum officinale,* and pot marigolds, which are annuals, in containers of their own. *Symphytum officinale* is the comfrey to use for home remedies, rather than the dwarf, variegated form, which has been planted here for decoration.

You will need
stone urn
crocks (broken terracotta pots)
horticultural grit
loam-based potting compost (soil mix)
soilless potting compost (growing medium)
trowel
watering can

Plants
Aloe vera
comfrey (Symphytum officinale *and dwarf variegated form*)
houseleek (Sempervivum tectorum)
pot marigold (Calendula officinalis)
yarrow (Achillea millefolium)

— Maintenance —
Do not overwater; allow the compost to get nearly dry before re-watering. Yarrow has a creeping root system and will need to be kept in check by thinning it out.

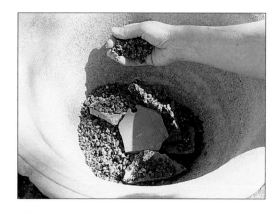

1 Position the pot before you start to fill it. Check that it has a large drainage hole and put in a layer of crocks (broken terracotta pots), topped with a layer of grit.

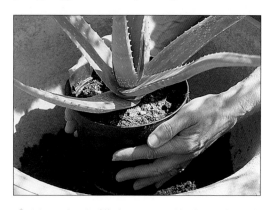

2 Two-thirds fill the pot with a loam-based potting compost (soil mix) mixed with a small amount of soilless compost (growing medium). Plant the aloe vera – leave it in its own pot, if you prefer, so that it can be removed easily before the first frosts. The yarrow can also be planted near the middle of the pot.

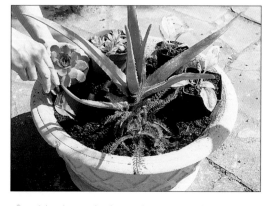

3 Plant houseleeks and variegated dwarf comfrey around the outside, filling in with extra compost as necessary. Water the plants in well.

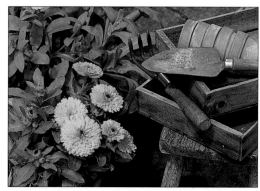

Above: Pot marigolds.

Opposite: Aloe vera *leaves contain a soothing gel. The plant makes a striking centrepiece in the container but as it is a tropical plant it doesn't tolerate frost and in cool climates can only be left outside in summer. Pot marigolds and comfrey are best grown in separate pots.*

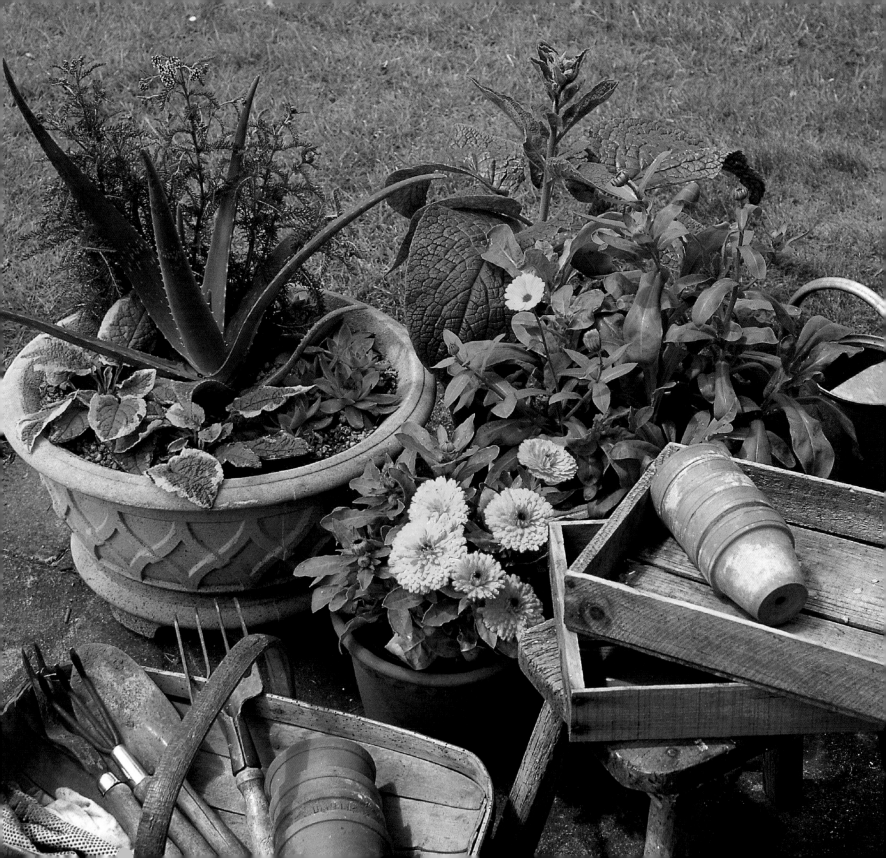

HERBS FOR HEALTHY HAIR

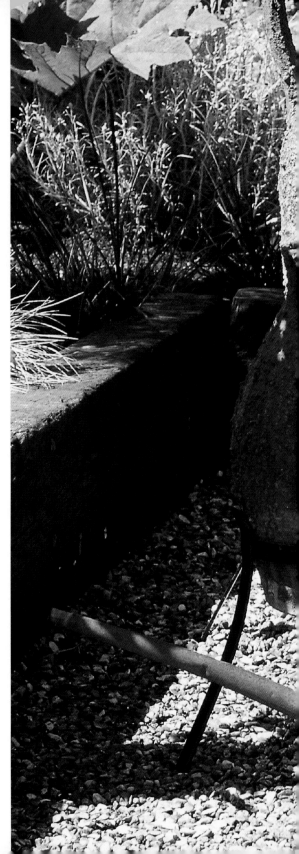

Making an infusion of fresh herbs for a hair rinse is as simple as brewing a cup of tea. Rosemary is the classic herb for dark hair, but its high essential oil content makes it a useful ingredient in a rinse for dry hair of any hue. Chamomile gives a sheen to fair hair, sage and southernwood help with dandruff and dry scalp problems, and lavender adds its inimitable scent to a rinse for any purpose.

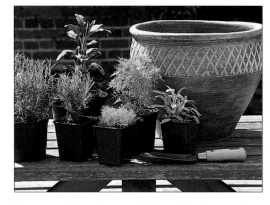

YOU WILL NEED
large container
crocks (broken terracotta pots)
potting compost (growing medium)
horticultural grit
trowel
watering can

PLANTS
double-flowered chamomile (Chamaemelum nobile *'Flore Pleno')*
lavender (Lavandula *'Hidcote'*, L. *'Munstead'*, L. stoechas)
rosemary (Rosmarinus officinalis) *upright and prostrate forms*
sage (Salvia officinalis)
golden sage (S. officinalis *'Icterina'*)
purple sage (S. officinalis purpurea)
southernwood (Artemisia abrotanum)

OPPOSITE: *Fresh herbs can be made into rinses to keep hair shiny and in tip-top condition. Grow them in an unusual pot to make an interesting focal point in the garden.*

1 Cover the drainage hole with a layer of crocks (broken terracotta pots). Fill to just below the rim with a gritty potting compost (growing medium). Firm it down gently.

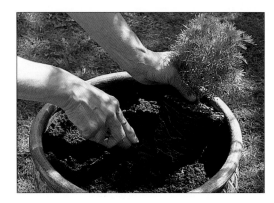

2 Tap each herb out of its pot in turn, make a hole in the compost with a trowel and press in the plant.

3 Once all the plants are in, fill in around them with extra compost as necessary and water them in thoroughly. Water and feed regularly and re-pot annually.

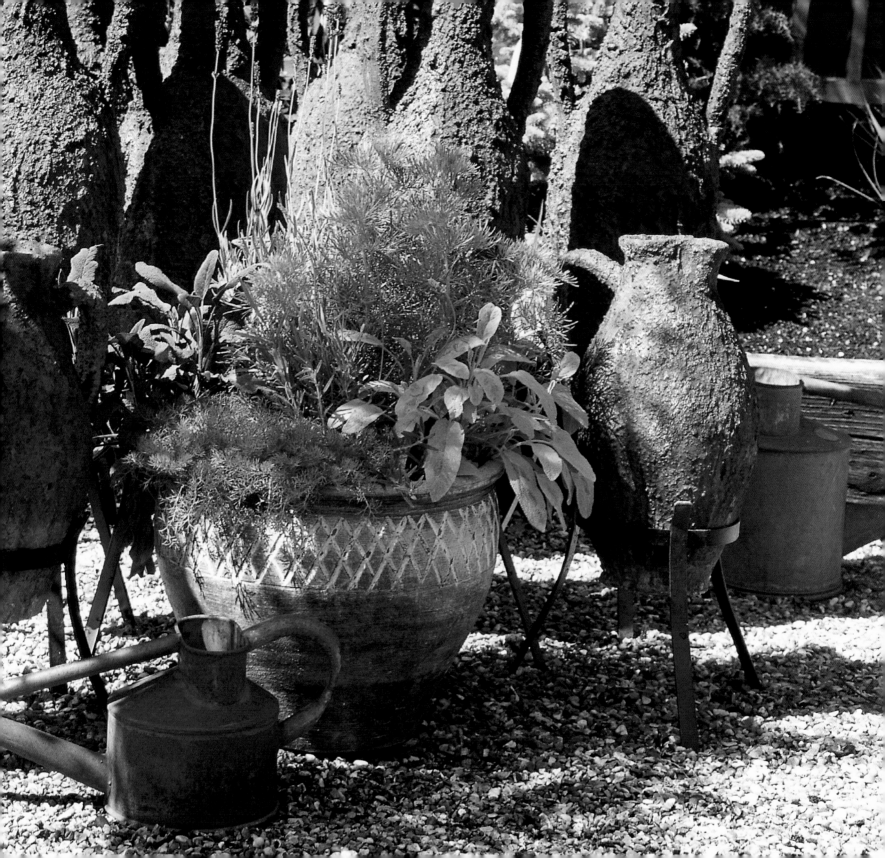

A TUSSIE-MUSSIE TO SOOTHE THE SENSES

That fragrance had the power to ward off disease was a widely held belief in days gone by. It was for this reason that people carried little bunches of herbs in crowded city streets – not just to guard against rotten smells, but to protect them from infection. It has been recorded that judges were provided with posies to avoid contracting gaol (jail) fever from prisoners brought to trial. The earliest tussie-mussies – the term can be traced back to at least 1440 – were simple bunches of sweet-smelling herbs tied with wool. They still make welcome gifts, especially for someone in hospital where formal florist's bouquets can be overpowering.

YOU WILL NEED
secateurs or scissors
fine florist's wire
raffia or coloured wool

PLANTS
Rosa gallica *'Rosa mundi'*
thyme (Thymus vulgaris)
cotton lavender (Santolina chamaecyparissus)
sage (Salvia officinalis)
southernwood (Artemisia abrotanum)
purple sage (S. officinalis purpurea)
rosemary (Rosmarinus officinalis)

— *TIP* —
You could also use lavender, scented-leaf pelargoniums, lemon verbena, bay, mint or marjoram.

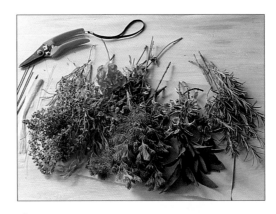

1 Before beginning the posy, assemble the plants and prepare the stems by stripping off the lower leaves and cutting them to even lengths. It is difficult to do this once you have started so prepare plenty in advance.

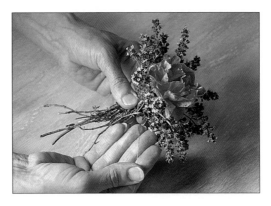

2 Start with the rose in the centre and surround it with flowering thyme, securing with a piece of florist's wire wound around the top of the stems. Take care to keep each new layer of herbs slightly below the previous one, so that the central bloom is not obscured.

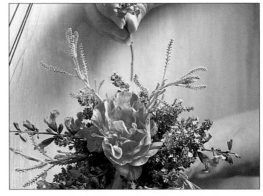

3 Build up the layers, adding circles of cotton lavender, sage flowers, southernwood, purple sage and rosemary. Keep the design symmetrical and fasten each layer with wire, as before.

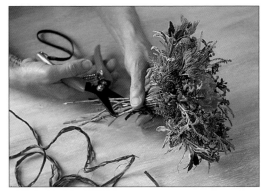

4 Cut all the stems to an even length and finish by binding them with raffia or coloured wool.

OPPOSITE: A traditional tussie-mussie is simple to put together with fragrant herbs picked from the garden and makes a welcome gift.

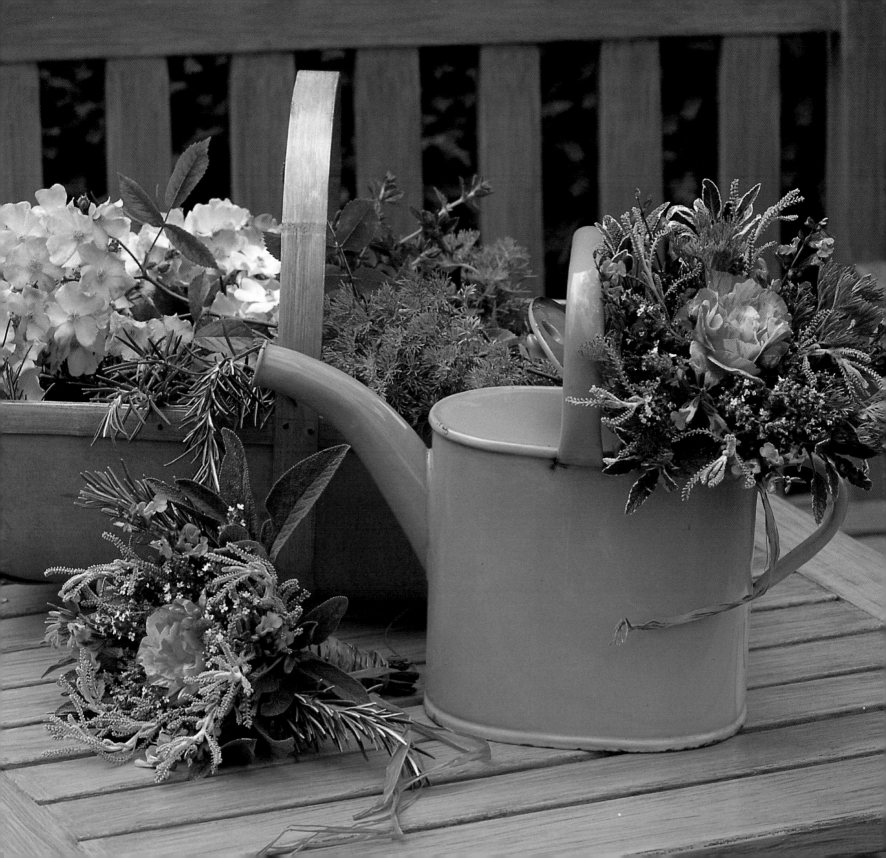

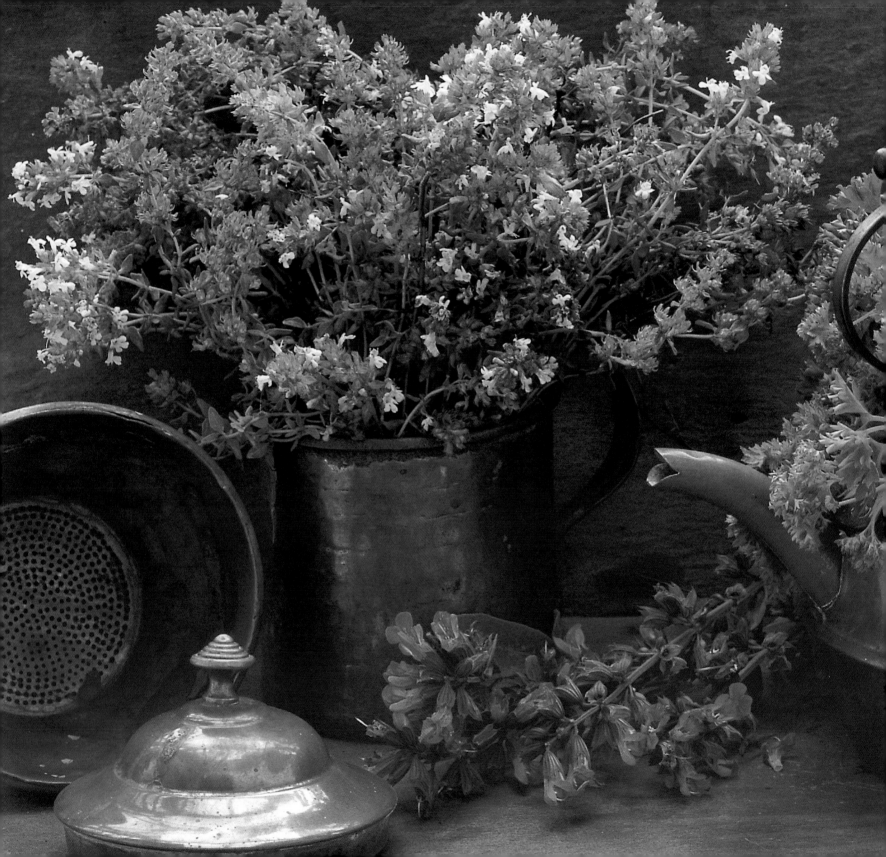

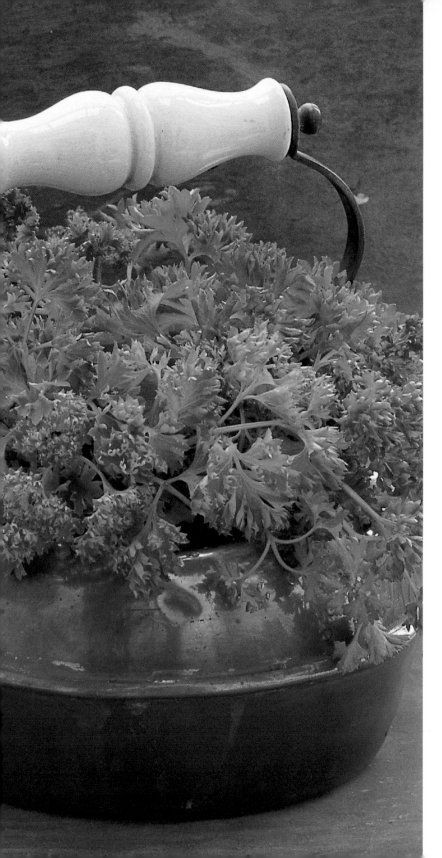

Chapter Two

Medicinal Herbs in Cookery, Tonics and Teas

"Let your medicine be your food – and your food your medicine."
Hippocrates

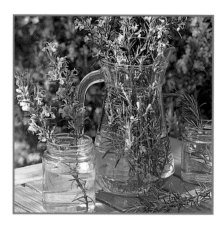

The emphasis in this chapter is on the therapeutic value of herbs taken internally, rather than on their general culinary uses. There are recipes for teas, vinegars, tinctures, tonics and other remedies, all to be taken in the small medicinal doses recommended. A nettle soup and some salads have also been included but here, too, their significance lies in the specific properties and actions of the herbs they contain.

Above: Rosemary makes a reviving tea and lends its bracing flavour to herb oils, tonic wine and dried herb seasoning.

Left: Familiar culinary herbs, thyme and sage, have antibacterial properties, while parsley is rich in vitamins and minerals.

41

HERBS AND SPICES IN A HEALTHY DIET

The connection between diet and health is undoubtedly important and herbs and spices have several key roles to play in this. Many of them have a direct medicinal action that can be taken into account when cooking with them. Garlic is thought to ward off colds and flu, lower cholesterol and reduce the risk of heart disease. Cayenne, with its antibacterial action, combats infections. Thyme, high in antioxidants, has been linked to slowing the ageing process, as well as having antiseptic properties. Pungent ginger counteracts nausea and aids the absorption of food.

It has been well documented that the consumption of certain foods boosts the immune system. The key is to eat plenty of fresh fruit, vegetables, whole grains and vegetable oils. This is because they contain antioxidants in the form of vitamins and minerals, which counteract the unstable and potentially harmful free radicals formed by the body's metabolism through stress, pollution and ageing.

RIGHT: Chopped herbs add flavour to bland, low-fat dishes.

BELOW: A flavoursome and health-giving bouquet garni *of fresh herbs.*

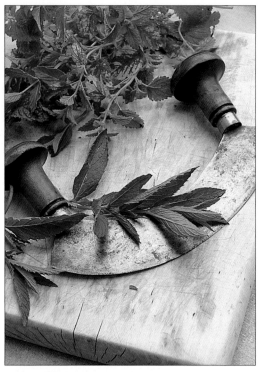

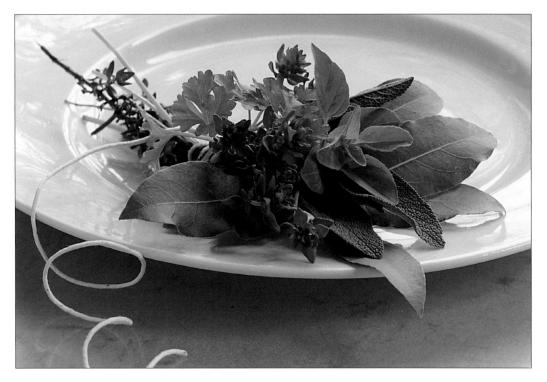

VITAMIN AND MINERAL PROPERTIES OF CULINARY HERBS

BORAGE: vitamin C, calcium, potassium.
CHICORY: potassium, B vitamins.
DANDELION: vitamin A, calcium, potassium, iron.
ELDERBERRIES: vitamins A, C.
GARLIC: vitamin C, potassium, selenium.
NETTLES: vitamins A, C, calcium, iron
PARSLEY: vitamins A, C, calcium, copper, iron, potassium.
WATERCRESS: vitamins A, B2, C, calcium.

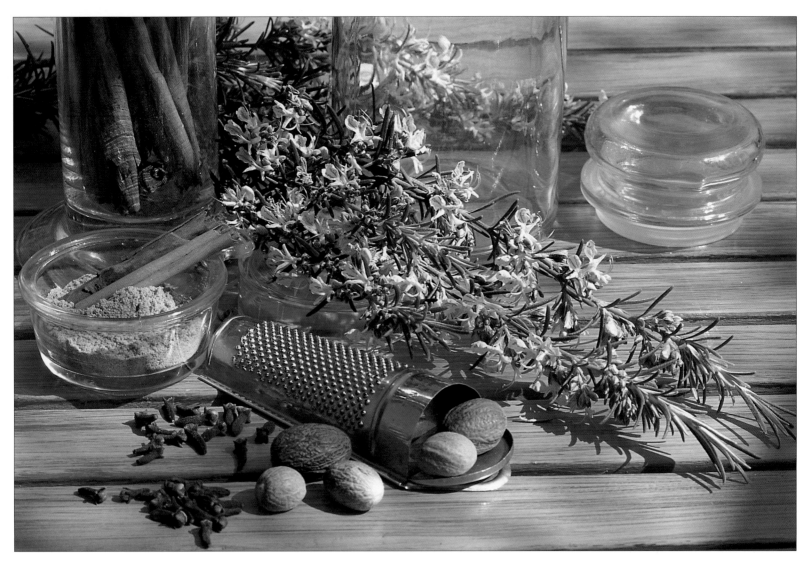

ABOVE: Herbs and spices in the diet stimulate gastric juices and act as digestives.

Herbs have a valuable contribution to make. Many contain these vital antioxidants, vitamins, minerals and trace elements. It is sometimes claimed that they are not eaten in large enough quantities to be worth counting, but this depends on whether you add herbs in token pinches or make them the main ingredient of a dish, as in a soup composed chiefly of nettles or a salad consisting primarily of dandelion leaves, parsley or watercress. There is also a cumulative effect; eat herbs every day and the benefits accrue. Herbs and spices are also well known for stimulating appetite and acting as digestives – fennel, dill and peppermint can all be put to good use here.

Apart from their intrinsic properties, herbs and spices are valuable in adding delicious flavours, especially important in a diet low in salt and fat which could otherwise taste bland. There are several ideas in the following pages for herbal seasonings to pep up recipes.

Finally, don't forget that food is there to be enjoyed – which in itself contributes to your general well-being.

HERB OILS

Vegetable oils are widely recognized as being a healthier addition to the diet than butter and other saturated animal fats. Flavoured with herbs, they add a new dimension to cooking. As well as tasting delicious, flavoured oils take on the properties of the herb and are important constituents of many healing remedies and natural beauty products.

Use a base oil which is not too strongly flavoured, such as sunflower, safflower or a light olive oil. Avoid cheap, blended vegetable oils. Use all oils in moderation, but never omit them from the diet, as they supply the body with essential fatty acids and help it to absorb vitamins A, D and E.

Basil Oil

Originating in India and widely grown in the Mediterranean, basil is an uplifting herb, prescribed by herbalists as an antidote to depression. It makes an excellent culinary oil for use in pasta dishes, pizzas or salad dressings.

INGREDIENTS
25g/1oz fresh basil leaves
300ml/1/2 pint/11/4 cups vegetable oil

—*TIP*—
It is best *not* to leave a sprig of the fresh herb in the finished oil, as after a week or so any leafy material will start to decay and adversely affect the keeping properties of the oil.

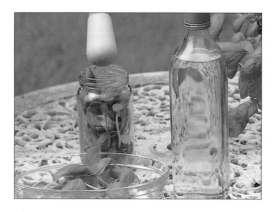

1 Wash the basil leaves if necessary and dry gently on kitchen paper (paper towel). Put them into a jar and crush them lightly to release the aroma of the essential oil.

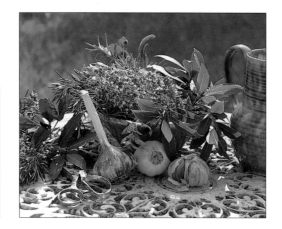

BELOW: Garlic is a first choice herb oil ingredient and is thought to ward off infections. Robustly flavoured herbs such as marjoram, thyme, rosemary, bay and sage make delicious herb oils. Use them singly or in combination.

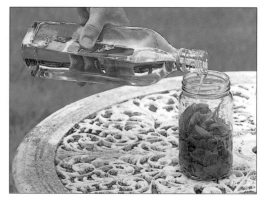

2 Fill the jar to the top with oil. Cover and leave in a warm place for one week.

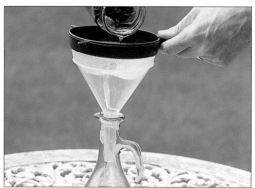

3 Strain off the basil leaves and pour the oil into a suitable bottle. (For a stronger flavour, put a fresh batch of leaves into the jar, pour the same oil in again, cover and leave for a further 5–7 days, then strain again.)

RIGHT: Vegetable oils suffused with herbs have many uses in natural remedies and a healthy diet. (LEFT TO RIGHT): Mixed Herb Oil, Cayenne and Garlic Oil, Basil Oil.

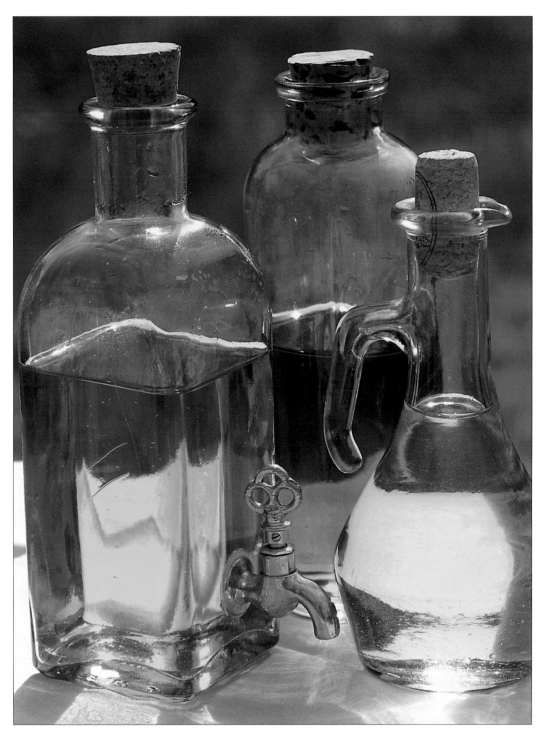

Follow the same method to flavour oil
with other herbs and spices. Marjoram,
thyme, rosemary, bay and sage are good
in combination, or could be used singly.
Cayenne and garlic are both antibacterial
and together make a richly flavoured oil
with a bit of a kick.

Mixed Herb Oil
INGREDIENTS
*equal quantities of fresh marjoram, thyme,
rosemary, bay and sage, about 40g/1½ oz
in all*
300ml/½ pint/1¼ cups vegetable oil

Cayenne and Garlic Oil
INGREDIENTS
10–15ml/2–3 tsp cayenne
4 crushed garlic cloves
300ml/½ pint/1¼ cups vegetable oil

BELOW: *The flavour of basil is notoriously
difficult to preserve when the herb is dried or
frozen, but a well-made basil oil retains all the
subtle flavour of the fresh herb.*

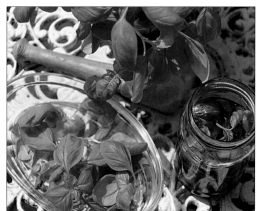

HERB VINEGARS

In cookery, herb vinegars give extra flavour to sauces and salad dressings, or an unusual piquancy to a compôte of fresh fruit. They also have valuable medicinal uses: they can be used as antiseptics for cleaning surfaces, or in compresses and poultices; some can be dabbed on to the skin to counteract a range of conditions from rashes to headaches, and others can be taken internally as a tonic or prophylactic. They are often used in beauty preparations too.

Cider vinegar is best for making herb vinegars, and many claims have been made for its health-giving properties. It restores the acid mantle of the skin and is a traditional ingredient in skin lotions and hair rinses. White wine vinegar is also acceptable, but malt vinegar, including the colourless one, is too harsh and strongly flavoured for herbal use.

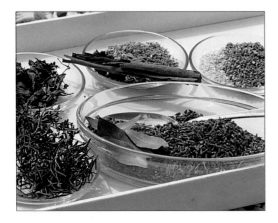

ABOVE: *Ingredients for Four Thieves Vinegar* (CLOCKWISE FROM RIGHT): *lavender and bay, rosemary, peppermint, cloves, cinnamon and wormwood, garlic and sage.*

Four Thieves Vinegar

During an outbreak of plague in medieval France, a gang of four thieves, who made a living by robbing the bodies of the dead, were said to avoid succumbing to the disease themselves by making liberal use of a strong herbal vinegar. Many versions of the recipe have been attributed to them. This formula, based on an amalgam of the old recipes, is effective as a mild antiseptic, or to take in prophylactic doses of 5ml/1 tsp, two or three times daily, when exposed to colds and other infections.

INGREDIENTS
*15ml/1 tbsp each dried lavender, rosemary,
sage and peppermint
2–3 bay leaves
10ml/2 tsp dried wormwood
5ml/1 tsp garlic granules
5ml/1 tsp ground cloves
5ml/1 tsp ground cinnamon
600ml/1 pint/2½ cups cider vinegar*

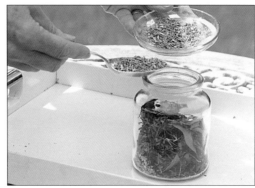

1 Put all the dry ingredients into a jar.

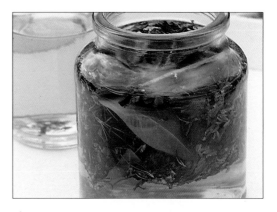

2 Fill the jar with cider vinegar. Cover tightly and leave in a warm place, such as a sunny windowsill or by a boiler, for 10 days.

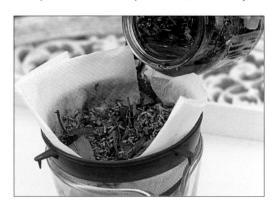

3 Strain off the vinegar, through a sieve lined with kitchen paper, into a clean jug, then pour it into a sterilized bottle and seal.

—CAUTION—
Do not take internally for longer than 2 weeks at a time. Do not take if pregnant, as wormwood is a uterine stimulant.

—*VARIATIONS*—

Follow the same method to make a range of other herb vinegars which have both culinary and medicinal uses.

Raspberry Vinegar

INGREDIENTS

115g/4oz raspberries
600ml/1 pint/2½ cups cider vinegar

CULINARY: Sprinkle over fruit salads or add to salad dressing.
MEDICINAL: Dilute in an equal quantity of warm water as a gargle for a sore throat.

Blackberry Vinegar

INGREDIENTS

115g/4oz blackberries
600ml/1 pint/2½ cups cider vinegar

CULINARY: Mix with salad oil as a dressing for apple coleslaw.
MEDICINAL: For arthritis or gout, stir 10–15ml/2–3 tsp into a small glass of hot, still mineral water with 5ml/1 tsp honey.

Rose Petal Vinegar

INGREDIENTS

50g/2oz fresh rose petals
600ml/1 pint/2½ cups cider vinegar

CULINARY: Sprinkle over cucumber salad with dill, or add to home-cooked beetroot.
MEDICINAL: Dip a cotton handkerchief into the vinegar and apply to the temples to ease a headache.

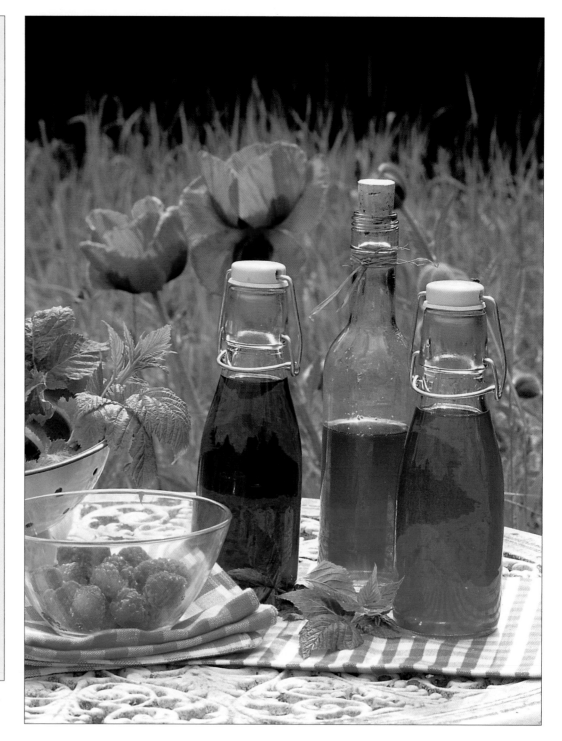

RIGHT (FROM LEFT TO RIGHT): *Blackberry, Four Thieves and Raspberry Vinegars.*

HERB TEAS

One of the easiest ways to benefit from the properties of a herb is to drink it as a tea, or tisane. Herbal infusions make wonderfully refreshing drinks and provide a caffeine-free alternative to ordinary tea and coffee. Many commercial brands are available but the taste of teas made from fresh or home-dried garden herbs is hard to beat and ensures maximum benefit from the properties of the plants.

If you are using fresh herbs, wash them first, especially if they have been picked from the wild. Allow 30ml/2 tbsp fresh or 15ml/1 tbsp dried herb to each 600ml/1pt/2½ cups water. To make a single cup, use two small sprigs of fresh or 5ml/1 tsp dried herb. Herb teas can be sweetened with honey to taste, but never add milk.

For medicinal purposes, take a cupful of the appropriate tea three times a day, and for sleep disturbances, drink a cup in the evening before going to bed. Chamomile is a favourite bed-time drink for its soothing action.

Cafetière method

A cafetière provides a convenient alternative to an ordinary teapot as it cuts out the need for straining.

—CAUTION—
Herbs are powerful. Do not make teas stronger or drink more frequently than recommended. Medical supervision is essential in pregnancy.

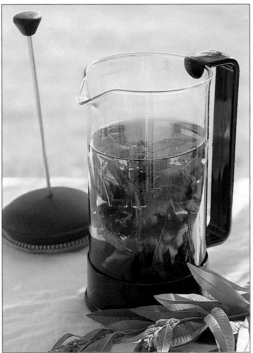

1 Put fresh or dried herbs (this is lemon verbena), in the quantities given above, into a warmed pot and pour on boiling water.

2 Replace the lid to prevent dissipation of the fragrant vapours, then leave to brew for 3–4 minutes.

3 Push down the plunger when the tea is strong enough to serve. Lemon verbena makes a refreshing tea-time drink.

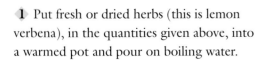

Tisanière Method

A traditional tisanière is a cup with an integral strainer and a lid to put on while the tea is brewing. This is very important, as it prevents the properties of the herb from evaporating in the steam and dissipating into the air.

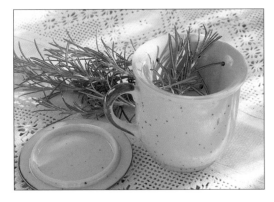

1 Put a sprig of herb (this is rosemary) into the strainer compartment of the tisanière and pour in boiling water.

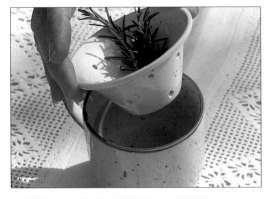

2 Put on the lid and leave to brew for 3–4 minutes. Lift out the strainer before drinking the tea.

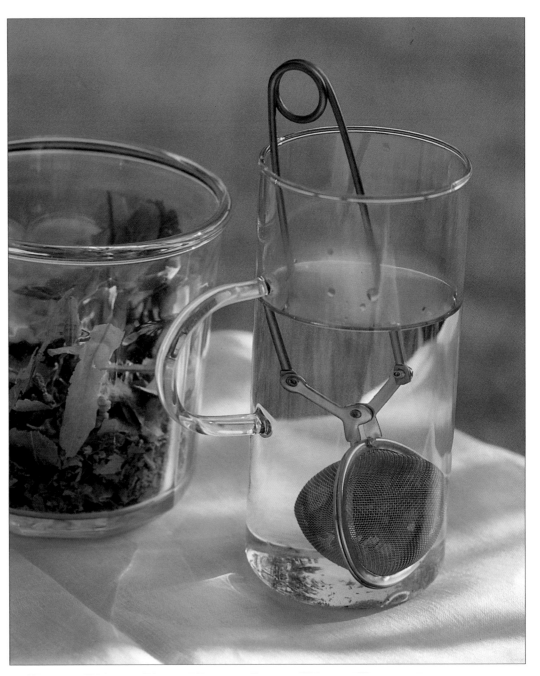

Above: A tea infuser, available from health or cookware stores, is a useful gadget for making a single cup of tea from dried herbs.

HERB TEAS FOR EVERYDAY PROBLEMS

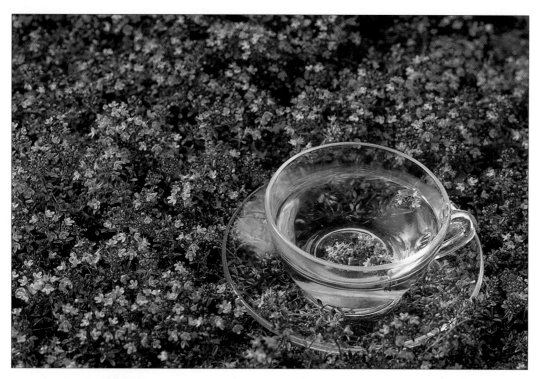

Teas for Coughs and Colds

PURPLE SAGE AND THYME: Use in equal quantities in a tea to ease a sore throat. For a more powerful effect, add 1.5ml/¼ tsp cayenne pepper, which has antibacterial properties.

PEPPERMINT, ELDERFLOWER, CHAMOMILE, AND LAVENDER: At the onset of a cold, use 2.5ml/½ tsp of each of the first three, with a pinch of lavender, per cupful of water. Add a sprinkling of ground ginger, 5ml/1 tsp honey and a slice of lemon.

HOREHOUND: Make with the fresh or dried herb. Sweeten to taste with honey and add a dash of lemon juice. Take it for a chesty cold.

ABOVE: The antiseptic and antibacterial properties of thyme make it a first-choice tea for sore throats, colds and chest infections.

HYSSOP: For a cough, use the fresh or dried leaf, or the leaf and flowers. Hyssop is quite bitter, so sweeten this tea with honey and a little freshly squeezed orange juice, which adds valuable vitamin C.

THYME: Its antiseptic properties are good for chest infections. Use 5ml/1 tsp dried thyme, or 10ml/2 tsp fresh, per cup. It has a warming effect and can also be used for digestive problems and stomach chills.

Teas for Digestive Troubles

CHAMOMILE: For digestive upsets, brew tea from the dried flowers. For a change, substitute half the chamomile for dried peppermint.

PEPPERMINT AND LEMON BALM: Use fresh herbs in equal quantities for a pleasantly flavoured digestive tea to drink after a meal.

DILL: Acts gently to ease indigestion and can be given to babies and young children. Allow 5ml/1 tsp lightly crushed dill seed to a cup of water and boil for 10 minutes. Strain and allow to cool before drinking.

FENNEL SEED: For flatulence and indigestion. Crush the seeds and simmer in an enamel saucepan for 10 minutes before straining. This is also a traditional slimming aid and can help relieve hunger pangs. Caraway seeds can be prepared in the same way or combined with fennel, in equal quantities.

BELOW: Fennel tea is made with the seeds of the herb. Take it for indigestion and as an aid to losing weight.

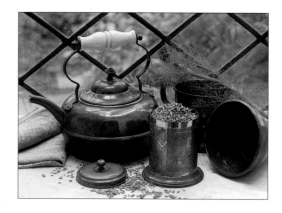

Tonic Teas

STINGING NETTLES: A tonic tea to cleanse the system. It may also help alleviate rheumatism and arthritic pains. Chop up a small handful of young, fresh nettle leaves and infuse in 600ml/1pint/2½ cups boiling water before straining.

SPEARMINT: The tea has a zingy, uplifting taste. Use 15ml/1 tbsp chopped fresh leaves per cup and sweeten to taste.

BASIL: Calming to the nervous system, it also helps relieve nausea. Add 3–4 fresh leaves per cup.

Early Morning Teas

LEMON VERBENA: The fresh or dried leaves make an uplifting drink with a lively flavour for waking up the system.

PEPPERMINT: Has a gently stimulating effect when taken first thing in the morning.

BELOW: Lemon balm makes a zingy "tonic" tea and is a traditional anti-depressant.

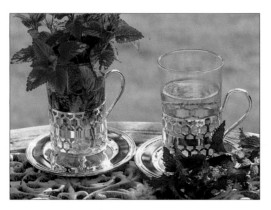

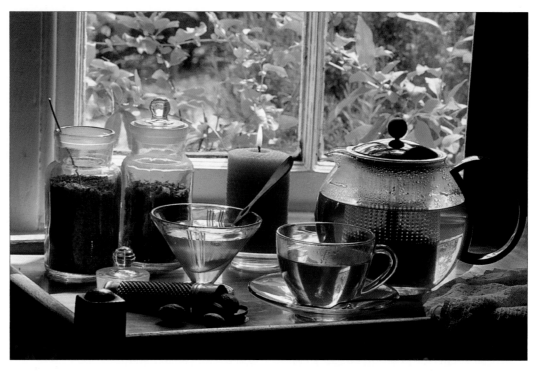

BERGAMOT: The leaves and flowers make a tea with a distinctive, scented taste that is very refreshing.

Teas for Disturbed Sleep

CHAMOMILE: One of the best bedtime drinks for those who have difficulty getting to sleep. It is calming to the nervous system, as well as a digestive. Make it with 5ml/1 tsp dried chamomile to a cup and try adding a pinch of lavender for extra relaxation.

LIMEFLOWER AND ELDERFLOWER: A pleasant bedtime tea. Add a dash of grated nutmeg and sweeten with honey.

VALERIAN: Use the dried and shredded root for a tea to calm the nerves. Using 10ml/2 tsp to a cup of water, simmer gently for 20 minutes in an enamel pan with a lid. Let it cool, then strain, re-heat and drink.

ABOVE: Limeflowers and elderflowers have a gentle soporific action as a night-time drink. Sweeten with honey to taste.

Teas for Headaches, Anxiety and Depression

ROSEMARY: One of the more pleasant tasting teas when made with the fresh herb. Put one or two small sprigs per person into a teapot or cup and add boiling water. Rosemary is invigorating and refreshing. It clears the head and helps to ease headaches. Add a few betony leaves to relieve nervous tension.

LEMON BALM: For tea, always use the freshly gathered herb. It has a long tradition as an anti-depressant.

ST JOHN'S WORT: Use fresh or dried leaves and flowers. It helps to relieve nervous tension, anxiety and depression.

ROSEMARY TONIC WINE

Rosemary has a long tradition of use as a "tonic" herb with a reputation for lifting the spirits. As Gerard declared, "Rosemary comforteth the heart and maketh it merrie". There is no better herb for infusing in a spiced wine to make a restorative pick-me-up. Originally found growing on the Mediterranean coast – the Latin name rosmarinus means "dew of the sea" – rosemary acts as a mild antidepressant and calms the nerves. Ginger and cloves are thought to boost the immune system and, along with cinnamon, aid digestion. Use a good quality wine for this recipe, as the addition of herbs cannot improve an inferior one. Drink half a small wineglassful (50ml/2 fl oz/¼ cup) not more than twice a day as a restorative when you are feeling tired and run-down.

INGREDIENTS
handful of fresh rosemary leaves
2 small cinnamon sticks
5 cloves
5ml/1 tsp ground ginger
grating of nutmeg
bottle of claret or other good quality red wine

—CAUTION—
Studies have shown that there are positive health benefits to drinking a glass of red wine daily, but beware of exceeding guidelines on safe limits for alcohol consumption.

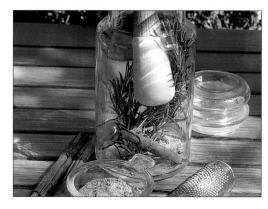

1 Put the rosemary, cinnamon sticks and cloves into a tall jar and crush them lightly, using a pestle to release their essential oils. Add the ginger and nutmeg.

2 Pour in the wine, seal the jar and leave it in a cool place for 7–10 days. Do not be tempted to leave it any longer than this as all the goodness will be extracted and the fresh plant material will begin to deteriorate.

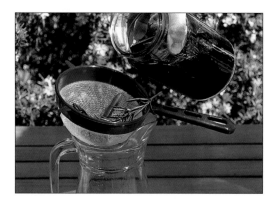

3 Strain off the wine into a jug and discard the rosemary.

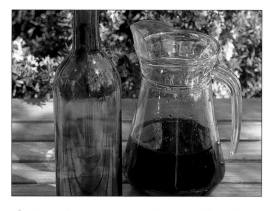

4 Pour the wine into a clean, sterilized bottle and seal with an airtight stopper or cork.

OPPOSITE: The refreshing taste and qualities of rosemary help to lift grey moods and mild depression. In folk tradition it is credited with improving memory.

—TO STERILIZE BOTTLES—
It is essential that bottles which are to contain wine – or any of the home-made preparations in this book – should be scrupulously clean. First wash them thoroughly in hot water, using a bottle brush. Then soak them in a sterilizing solution (as for babies' bottles) according to the manufacturer's instructions, or immerse them in water in a large preserving pan, bring to the boil and simmer for 10 minutes. Allow to dry naturally or, more effectively, in a barely warm oven.

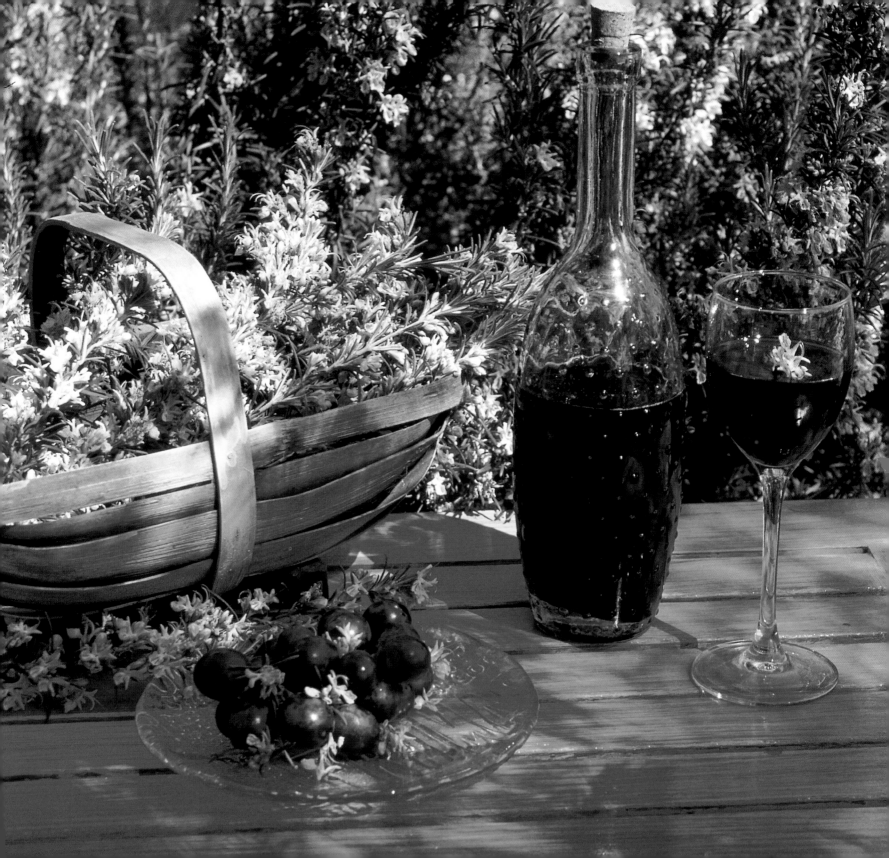

SPRING TONIC SOUP

The consumption of nettles as a springtime tonic goes back many centuries. Nettles are rich in iron, contain calcium and other minerals, and vitamins A and C. Research studies show that nettle extract helps to flush away uric acid, an excess of which causes arthritis.

Chicken stock is not essential – you can use water or vegetable stock instead – but it has long been claimed to be a mild antibiotic and it is helpful if you are fighting a viral infection.

INGREDIENTS
large handful of nettle tops
25g/1oz/2 tbsp butter or margarine
1 onion, chopped
2 garlic cloves, crushed
450g/1lb potatoes, peeled and diced
5–6 juniper berries, crushed
25g/1oz parsley
600ml/1 pint/2¹/2 cups home-made chicken stock
600ml/1 pint/2¹/2 cups milk
salt, pepper and cayenne pepper
yogurt or fromage frais, to serve

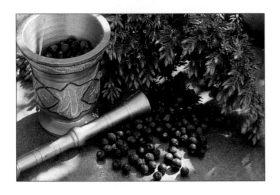

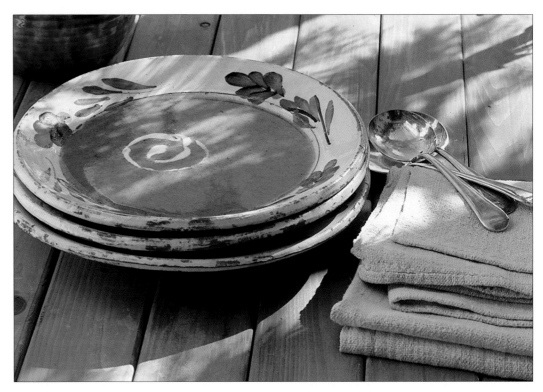

1 Wearing rubber gloves, pick the young central nettle leaves from the tip of each plant.

2 Melt the butter or margarine and add the onion, garlic, potatoes and crushed juniper berries. Cook gently for 4–5 minutes.

3 Stir in the nettle tops and parsley and cook for a further minute until they have wilted. Add the stock and simmer for about 15 minutes, until the potatoes are tender.

4 Blend in a food processor or blender until smooth. Return the soup to the rinsed-out pan and stir in the milk. Reheat gently, season to taste with salt, pepper and cayenne and serve, adding a swirl of yogurt or fromage frais to each bowl.

ABOVE: Young nettle tops make a delicious tonic soup with a refreshing, lemony flavour.

LEFT: Juniper berries enhance the flavour of Spring Tonic Soup, and may help to ease arthritic pain.

SEASONINGS

If you are trying to cut down on your intake of fat and salt, herb and spice seasonings are a healthy alternative way to add extra flavour to food. Mix dried herbs into soups and casseroles, stir-fries and pasta sauces, or sprinkle them over lightly cooked vegetables. Nothing beats fresh herbs as seasoning. Tie them in small, mixed bunches and use as required as a *bouquet garni*.

Herbal Seasoning

Make this with home-grown and dried herbs, prepared in early summer when the fresh material is plentiful.

INGREDIENTS
DRIED HERBS: *lovage, marjoram, summer or winter savory, parsley, bay leaves, sage, thyme, rosemary*

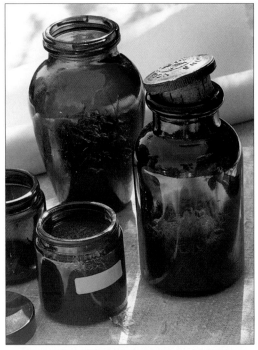

Hot and Spicy Seasoning

All these spices stimulate the appetite as well as acting as digestives. Cayenne and ginger help to boost circulation, and cayenne is antibacterial.

INGREDIENTS
GROUND SPICES: *mace, coriander, ginger, cayenne pepper*
freshly grated nutmeg

Mix together equal quantities of mace, coriander and ginger with one-third as much cayenne pepper and nutmeg. Store in a dark glass jar.

Left: Dark glass jars preserve the quality of dried herbs. Dried herbs will keep for up to a year if stored in a cool, dark place.

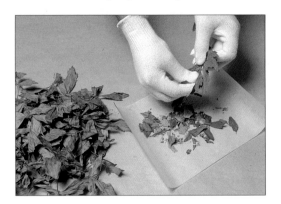

1 Crumble equal quantities of lovage, marjoram, summer or winter savory and parsley, with half as much bay leaf, sage and thyme. Cotton gloves will protect your fingers.

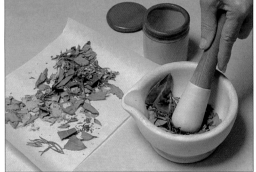

2 Pound the mixture in a bowl or with a mortar and pestle until reduced to a fine texture. Pour into airtight jars to store.

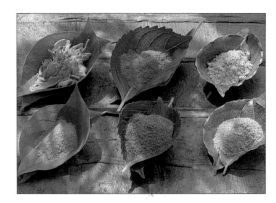

ABOVE: *Spices make a healthy addition to the diet. They have many attributes, from stimulating the appetite to boosting circulation.*

HERB AND FLOWER SALADS

Salads are an essential part of a healthy diet, and are especially nutritious when they include lavish quantities of fresh herbs. Try new and unusual combinations to add colour and variety to meals.

Dandelion Vitality Salad

Dandelion leaves are rich in potassium, iron and other minerals as well as vitamins A, B, C and D. Many herbalists use them to stimulate the liver, aid digestion and combat fluid retention, and they have a reputation for lifting the spirits into the bargain.

INGREDIENTS
1 yellow pepper
mixed salad leaves: dandelion, baby spinach,
rocket (arugula), lamb's lettuce (corn salad)
small bunch of spearmint
a few lemon balm leaves
borage flowers
pot marigold petals
vinaigrette dressing, to serve

Slice the pepper and mix it with the salad leaves in a large bowl. Snip in the mint and lemon balm, and top with borage flowers and marigold petals. Toss the salad gently in a vinaigrette dressing just before serving.

RIGHT: Dandelion salad is packed with vitamins and minerals to promote vitality.

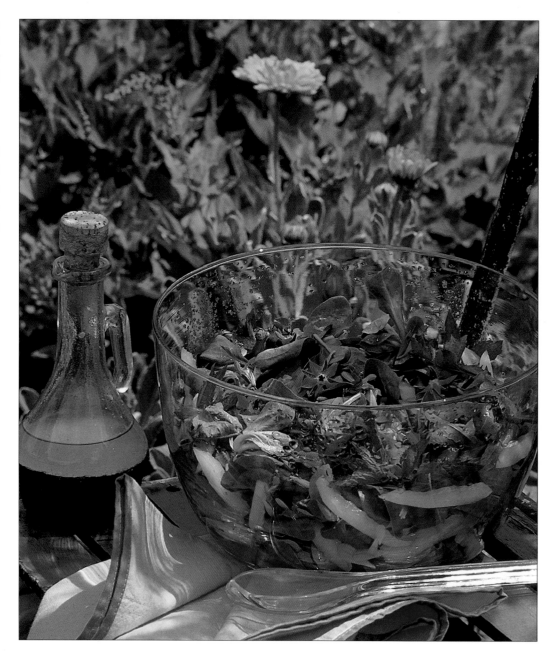

Nasturtium and Watercress Salad

Peppery nasturtium leaves contain vitamin C and the flowers are also edible, with a milder taste. Mix them with watercress and parsley, which both contain vitamins A, B and C, calcium, iron and other trace minerals, to make an energizing salad to help boost the immune system. Serve with orangeflower dressing.

INGREDIENTS
6–8 nasturtium flowers and leaves
bunch of watercress, stalks trimmed
25g/1oz flat-leaved and curly parsley, chopped
lettuce leaves
cucumber slices
1 large orange, peeled, sliced and cut in quarters
orangeflower dressing

1 Reserve some nasturtium flowers for decoration. Separate the petals of the rest and put them in a salad bowl with the watercress.

2 Shred the nasturtium leaves and add them to the salad, with the other ingredients. Toss with Orangeflower Dressing and garnish with nasturtium flowers.

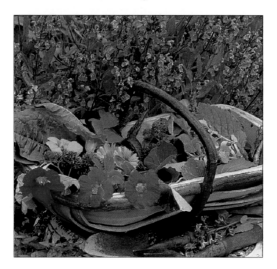

RIGHT: A basket of freshly gathered herbs and flowers provides wholesome ingredients for salads.

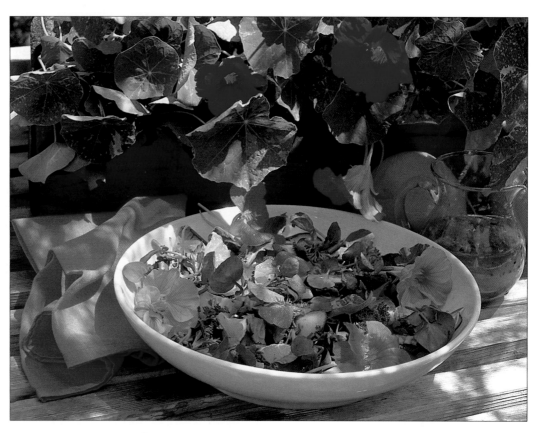

ABOVE: Nasturtiums make a cheerful addition to a watercress and orange salad.

Orangeflower Dressing

Orangeflower water has soothing properties and is a by-product of the steam distillation of neroli oil, a natural antidepressant.

INGREDIENTS
2.5ml/½ tsp garlic salt
5ml/1 tsp French mustard
45ml/3 tbsp safflower oil
15ml/1 tbsp orangeflower water
5ml/1 tsp lemon juice
small bunch of chives, finely snipped
freshly ground black pepper

Put all the ingredients in a screw-topped jar and shake thoroughly to mix before use.

GARLIC COLD SYRUP

The health-giving properties of garlic have been recognized since ancient Egyptian times when it was thought to bestow strength. Greek and Roman physicians prescribed it for respiratory infections and modern research confirms that garlic has antibacterial properties. It is also antiviral, a decongestant and may help the body combat infection. Combine it with honey, which is soothing and mildly antiseptic, in a syrup to prevent or relieve the symptoms of colds and flu. Take 10–15ml/2–3 tsp three times a day.

INGREDIENTS
1 head of garlic
300ml/½ pint/1¼ cups water
juice of ½ lemon
30ml/2 tbsp honey

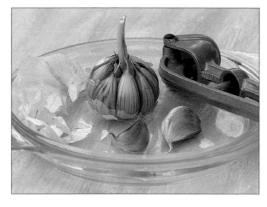

ABOVE: *"Garlic … a remedy for all diseases and hurts."* NICOLAS CULPEPER, COMPLETE HERBAL *(1653).*

RIGHT: *Garlic Syrup is a useful standby for combating infections. Take it at the first sign of a cold.*

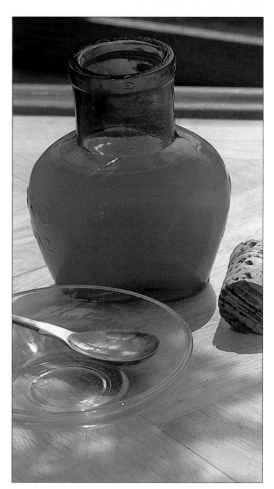

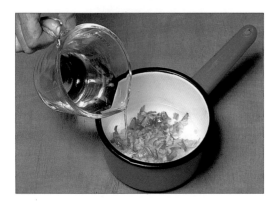

1 Crush the garlic cloves – there is no need to peel them – and put them in a pan with the water. Bring to the boil and simmer gently for 20 minutes.

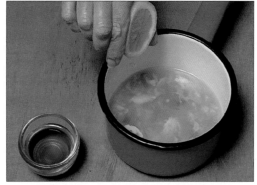

2 Add the lemon juice and honey and simmer for a further 2–3 minutes. Allow the mixture to cool slightly, then strain it into a clean, dark glass jar or bottle with an airtight lid. Keep for 2–3 weeks in the refrigerator.

FRUIT CORDIALS AND SYRUPS

There is a freshness and intensity of flavour in home-made cordials that is very rarely present in their commercial counterparts. They will keep from year to year and can be used for flavourings for ice creams and sorbets as well as making delicious drinks.

Elderflower and Lime Cordial

Elderflowers, which are anticatarrhal, and limes with their high vitamin C content, make an effectively soothing drink for summer colds.

INGREDIENTS
10 fresh elderflower heads
2–3 limes, sliced
675g/1½ lb/3 cups sugar
5ml/1 tsp citric acid
5ml/1 tsp cream of tartar
1 litre/1¾ pints/4 cups boiling water

1 Wash and pick over the elderflowers thoroughly. Put them into a large bowl with the sliced limes. Add the sugar, citric acid and cream of tartar. Set aside for 2 hours.

2 Pour in the boiling water and leave to stand for 24 hours. Strain the syrup into sterilized bottles and cork. The cordial will keep, chilled, for 2–3 months. To serve, dilute with about twice as much water.

RIGHT: Elderflower cordial makes a soothing drink for summer rhinitis and hayfever.

Elderberry Rob

Elderberries are rich in vitamins A and C and contain bioflavonoids, which give support to the immune system. Take the syrup with lemon juice, diluted to taste in hot water, for a feverish cold. The syrup keeps for several months.

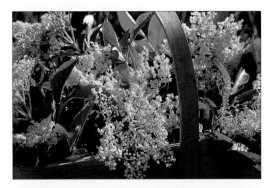

INGREDIENTS
1kg/2¼ lb elderberries
350g/12oz/1½ cups sugar
grated rind and juice of 1 orange
10 coriander seeds
1 cinnamon stick

Put all the ingredients into a pan and heat gently until the sugar is dissolved. Simmer for about 20 minutes. Strain and bottle.

LEFT: Make the most of an abundance of elderflowers: cook them with gooseberries and soft fruit, add to tinctures and lotions, or dry them for winter use and in teas.

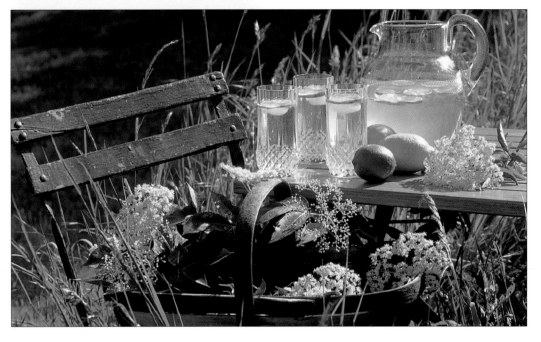

COUGH AND COLD DECOCTIONS

A decoction is made by simmering herbal ingredients in water. It is often used for roots and barks, which need cooking to extract their vital properties.

Ginger and Lemon Decoction for Sore Throats

Ginger is warming and stimulating and encourages sweating to eliminate toxins and dispel mucus and catarrh. This decoction will keep for 2–3 days.

INGREDIENTS
115g/4oz piece of fresh root ginger
600ml/1 pint/2½ cups water
juice and rind of 1 lemon
pinch of cayenne pepper

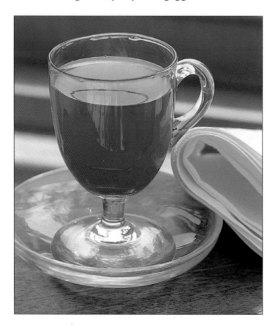

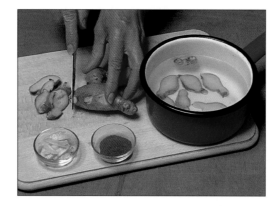

1 Slice the ginger root – there's no need to peel it – and put it in a pan with the water, lemon rind and cayenne.

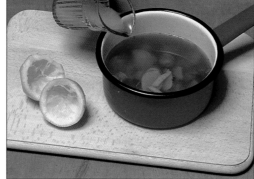

2 Bring to the boil, cover the pan and simmer for 20 minutes. Remove from the heat and add the lemon juice. Drink a small cupful at a time, sweetened with honey to taste.

LEFT: *A decoction of ginger and lemon relieves the discomfort of a sore throat.*

RIGHT: *Lemons with fresh ginger.*

Thyme and Borage Cough Linctus

Borage was traditionally used in cough syrup recipes, and thyme has antiseptic properties.

INGREDIENTS
25g/1oz fresh or 15g/½ oz dried thyme
25g/1oz fresh or 15g/½ oz dried borage
flowers and leaves
2 x 5cm/2in cinnamon sticks
600ml/1 pint/2½ cups water
juice of 1 small lemon
100g/4oz/½ cup honey

1 Put the herbs into a pan with the cinnamon and water. Bring to the boil, cover with a lid and simmer for 20 minutes. Strain off the herbs and return the liquid to the pan. Simmer, uncovered, until reduced by half.

2 Add the lemon juice and honey and simmer gently for 5 minutes. Bottle and store in a cool place. Bottled, it will keep for at least 2 months. Take 5ml/1 tsp, as required.

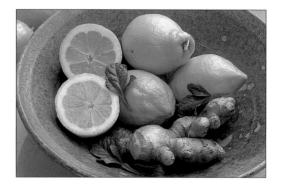

SORE THROAT GARGLES

Gargling with an infusion of fresh herbs can ease the discomfort of a sore throat. When fresh herbs are not available, dried ones can be substituted, using 30ml/2 tbsp in 600ml/1 pint/2½ cups water.

Thyme and Sage Gargle
Gargle with this mixture at the first sign of a sore throat. It can also be taken internally, 10ml/2 tsp at a time, 2–3 times a day. Use up within a week.

INGREDIENTS
*small handful each of fresh sage and thyme
leaves
600ml/1 pint/2½ cups boiling water
30ml/2 tbsp cider vinegar
10ml/2 tsp honey
5ml/1 tsp cayenne pepper*

1 Put the roughly chopped leaves into a jug, pour in the boiling water, cover and leave for 30 minutes.

2 Strain off the leaves and stir in the cider vinegar, honey and cayenne.

ABOVE: Fresh thyme and sage are the raw ingredients for an antiseptic gargle to ease a sore throat.

RIGHT: Horehound (with silvery leaves) combines well with aromatic hyssop (with blue flowers) for a gargle to combat a cough.

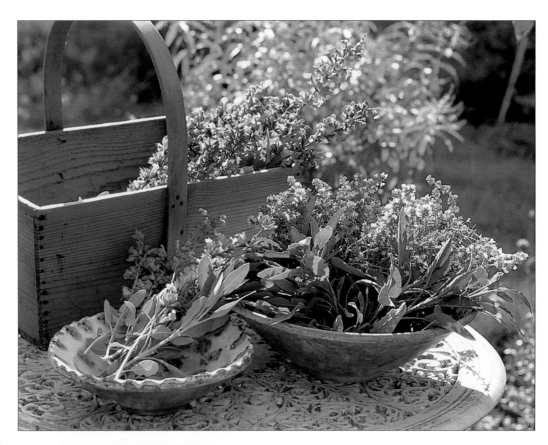

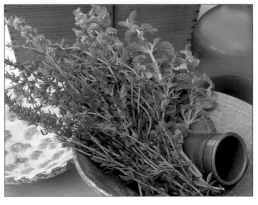

Hyssop and Horehound Gargle
Both hyssop and white horehound have long been considered by herbalists through the ages to be effective remedies in the treatment of coughs. They also combine well to make a strong gargle. Make an infusion of the leaves and flowering tops from both herbs, following the directions given for Thyme and Sage Gargle. Sipping herb teas can bring relief for a sore throat.

TINCTURES

Tinctures are an effective way to extract the active ingredients of plants. They can be made with fresh or dried plant material steeped in a mixture of alcohol and water. Vodka is the most suitable alcohol, since it is a pure spirit containing few additives. Tinctures will keep for up to two years as the alcohol acts as a preservative. Take no more than 5ml/1 tsp, 3–4 times a day, diluted in a little water or fruit juice, if preferred. Tinctures can also be applied externally, by adding them to liniments, compresses and other preparations.

Lavender Tincture

The following recipe can be adapted to make other tinctures using dried herbs.

INGREDIENTS
15g/¹/2 oz dried lavender
250ml/8 fl oz/1 cup vodka, made up to
300ml/¹/2 pint/1¹/4 cups with water

> —*TIP*—
> Dark glass bottles prevent deterioration of the contents by light. If you do use clear glass, keep the tinctures in a dark cupboard.

> —*CAUTION*—
> Under no circumstances use industrial alcohol, methylated or white spirits for tinctures, as they are highly toxic.

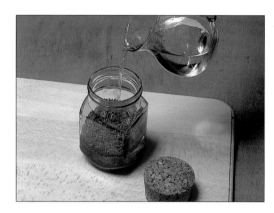

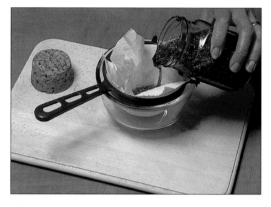

1 Put the dried lavender into a glass jar and pour in the vodka and water mixture. It will almost immediately start to turn a beautiful lavender blue.

3 Strain off the lavender through a sieve lined with kitchen paper (paper towel) before pouring into a sterilized glass bottle. Seal with a cork and store for future use.

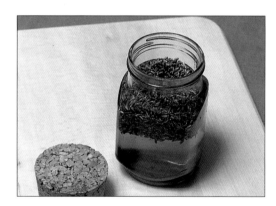

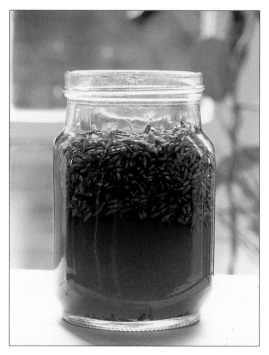

2 Put a lid on the jar and leave in a cool, dark place for 7–10 days (no longer), shaking occasionally. The tincture turns dark purple.

RIGHT: The active properties of lavender are extracted as the tincture turns from palest blue to dark purple. Strain off the flowers before they begin to deteriorate.

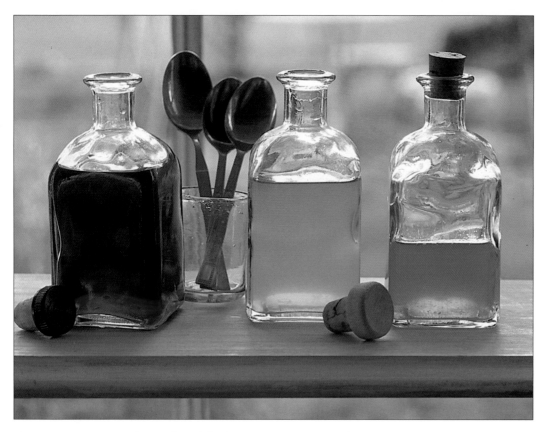

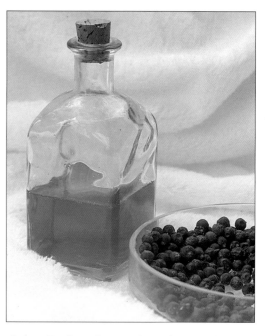

ABOVE: *Juniper tincture is made from the dried berries.*

ABOVE: LEFT TO RIGHT: *Lavender, violet leaf and juniper tinctures.*

BELOW: *Fresh raspberry leaves make a tincture for the relief of mouth ulcers.*

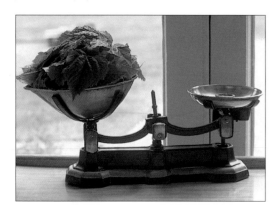

Raspberry Leaf Tincture

Use these proportions for other tinctures made with fresh plant material.

INGREDIENTS

50g/2 oz fresh raspberry leaves, coarsely chopped
250ml/8 fl oz/1 cup vodka, made up to 300ml/1/2 pint/1 1/4 cups with water

Follow the method for making lavender tincture. If the liquid does not quite cover the leaves, top up with a little extra vodka and water. Fresh leaves soak up more liquid, so squeeze them out well by pressing with a wooden spoon when straining.

—*TINCTURES AND THEIR USES*—
LAVENDER: For headaches, nervous disorders and depression. Take diluted, or add to a compress.
RASPBERRY LEAF: For mouth ulcers and inflamed gums. Dilute in an equal quantity of warm water and use as a mouthwash.
JUNIPER: For rheumatism. Add it to a liniment for aching joints.
ELDERFLOWER: For colds and hayfever. Make it with the dried flower. Take early in the season, before pollen counts rise, for hayfever.
VIOLET: For insomnia. Make with the flowers of sweet violet (*Viola odorata*).

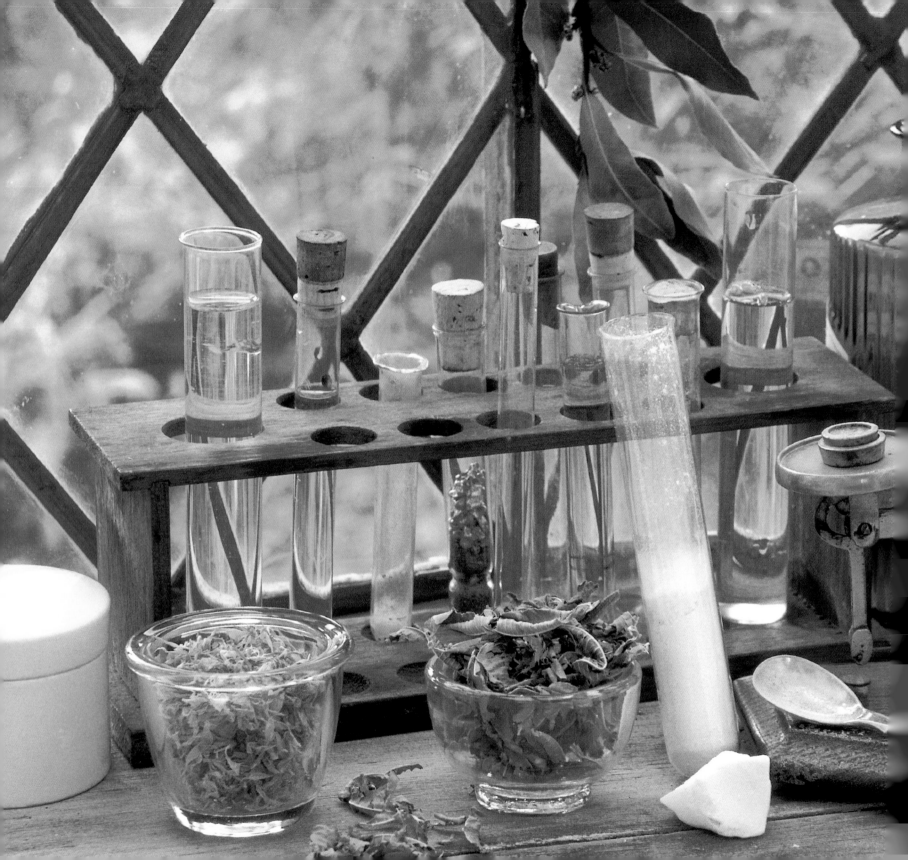

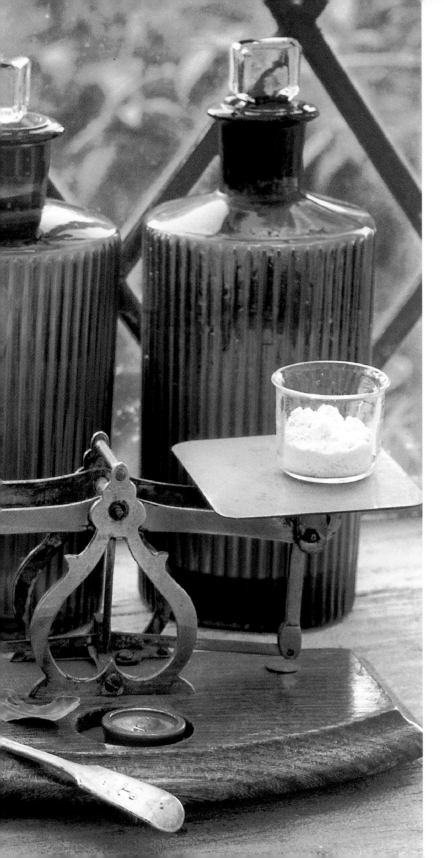

CHAPTER THREE

AROMATIC REMEDIES, SALVES AND LOTIONS

"Bring forth healthfull Hearbes for to heale many diseases."
NICOLAS MONARDES, *JOYFULL NEWES OUT OF THE NEWE FOUNDE WORLDE* (1569)

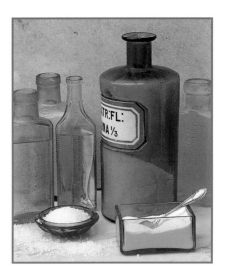

This chapter describes preparations to apply externally to the body – lotions, rubs, ointments and poultices. It also suggests ways you can benefit from the powerful aromatic properties of herbs by inhaling their fragrance through steam, or by making them into pillows and sachets.

ABOVE AND LEFT: Dried herbs and other ingredients for making healing preparations at home.

65

FIRST AID FOR THE SKIN

Freshly picked herbs and kitchen ingredients can be put to use as first aid for insect bites and stings, minor burns, bruises and grazes (scrapes). It is also helpful to buy a few simple preparations to keep in the medicine cupboard for such eventualities.

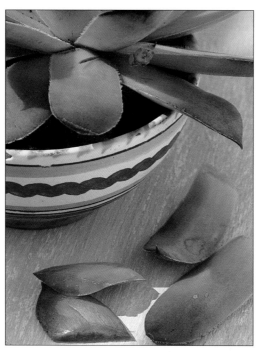

*Above: Houseleek (*Sempervivum tectorum*) makes a handy first aid treatment.*

Left: Aloe vera, used in many commercial products, is renowned for its healing properties.

Right: Raw onion is applied to relieve itching.

—ESSENTIAL OIL REMEDIES—

LAVENDER ESSENTIAL OIL: Dab lavender oil, diluted 1:5 in a little sunflower or almond oil, on minor burns, bites, bruises, or skin blemishes. Good quality pure lavender oil can also be used undiluted on the skin.

TEA TREE OIL: Make use of its antiseptic properties by diluting it in a little carrier oil and applying it to cuts and grazes once they have been cleaned.

—PLANT REMEDIES—

ALOE VERA OR HOUSELEEK: Break off a leaf of either plant, slit it open with a sharp knife and apply the gel that seeps out to minor burns, scalds, sunburn, bruises and bites.

LEMON BALM OR BASIL: Break off a handful of the fresh leaves of either plant to rub over insect bites.

DOCK LEAF: Rub nettle stings with a fresh dock leaf for immediate relief.

ONION: Cut in half or into thick slices, and apply to insect bites and bee stings. Freshly cut onion also reduces the itching of chilblains.

GARLIC: Peel and crush the cloves to apply to infected spots and pustules.

—STANDBY REMEDIES—

DISTILLED WITCH HAZEL: Apply on cotton wool to minor burns, sunburn, insect bites, cuts and bruises.

ARNICA CREAM: Rub gently on to bruises and sprains. Do not use on broken skin.

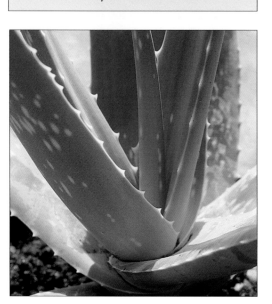

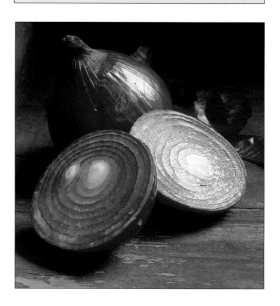

LAVENDER LIP BALM

It is quite simple to make your own sooth-ing cream for lips chapped by sun, wind, weather or illness. Beeswax and cocoa butter are rich emollients; wheatgerm oil, with its high vitamin E content, is a powerful antioxidant and lavender essential oil is well known for its healing ability. You can also apply a simple mixture of honey and rosewater as a salve for sore or chapped lips.

INGREDIENTS
5ml/1 tsp beeswax
5ml/1 tsp cocoa butter
5ml/1 tsp wheatgerm oil
5ml/1 tsp almond oil
3 drops lavender essential oil

RIGHT: Lavender lip balm is a rich and soothing salve for sore lips.

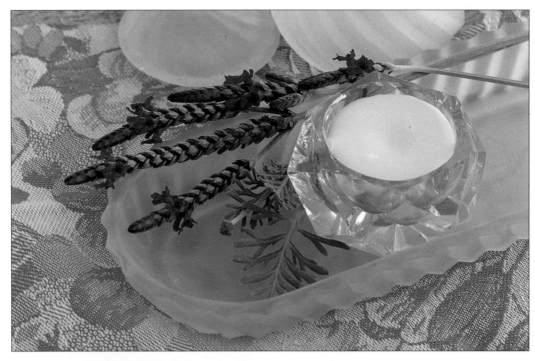

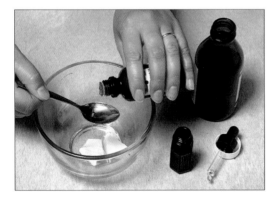

1 Put all the ingredients, except the laven-der essential oil, into a small bowl.

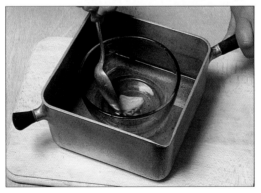

2 Set the bowl over a pan of simmering water and stir the contents until the wax has melted. Beeswax has a high melting point, so be patient.

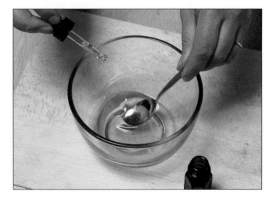

3 Remove from the heat and allow the mix-ture to cool for a few minutes before mixing in the lavender oil. Pour into a small jar and leave to set.

MARIGOLD SKIN SALVE

The bright orange flowers of pot marigolds (*Calendula officinalis*) have been valued by herbalists through the centuries for their healing properties. Gerard described them as being in such demand "to put into broths, in Physicall potions and for divers other purposes…that in some Grocers or Spice-sellers houses are to be found barrels filled with them." Today, calendula cream is recognized for its ability to soothe all manner of skin irritations, from insect bites and sunburn to eczema and other itchy rashes brought on by allergic reactions.

Calendula oil – which you can buy from specialist outlets – can be omitted, but it adds to the therapeutic action of the cream. Tincture of benzoin is an antiseptic and preservative.

INGREDIENTS

300ml/½ pint/1¼ cups boiling water
15g/½ oz dried pot marigold petals or
30g/1oz fresh petals
60ml/4 tbsp emulsifying ointment
15ml/1 tbsp glycerine
4 drops tincture of benzoin
4–5 drops calendula oil

RIGHT: *According to Macer's Herbal, just to look on marigold flowers is enough to draw "wicked humours" out of the head.*

OPPOSITE: *Pot marigolds make a wonderfully soothing and healing cream for minor skin irritations.*

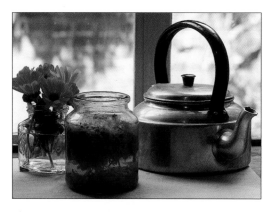

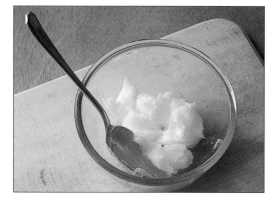

1 First make a strong marigold infusion by pouring the boiling water over the marigold petals in a jar. Cover and leave until cool before straining.

2 Put the emulsifying ointment and glycerine in a bowl set over a pan of gently simmering water and stir until melted. It will take about 10 minutes to melt.

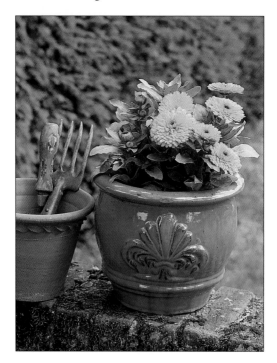

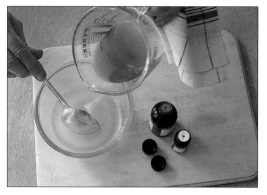

3 Remove from the heat and mix in 150ml/¼ pint/⅔ cup of the marigold infusion, with the tincture of benzoin and calendula oil. Stir the mixture until it has cooled and reached a consistency similar to double (heavy) cream. Pour into a small jar before it has thickened and set. It will keep for at least 6 months.

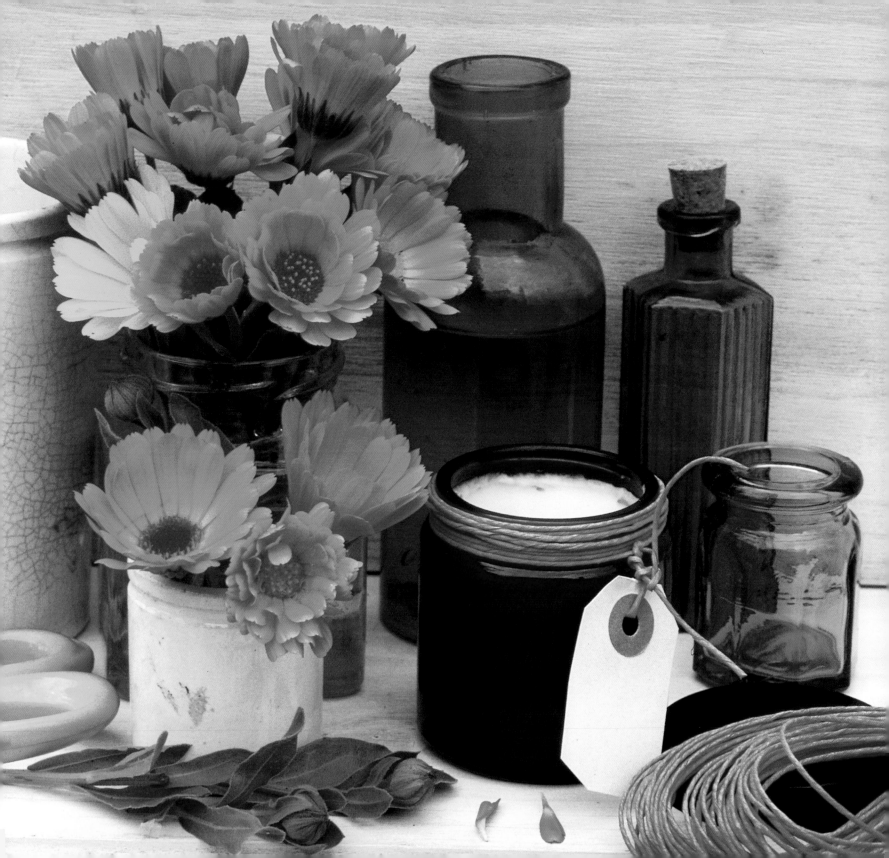

COMFREY BRUISE OINTMENT

Ointments are made from oils or fats with no water added. They form a protective layer over the skin rather than blending into it as would a cream. Petroleum jelly or paraffin wax make a more pleasant, longer-lasting base than the animal fats once used for the purpose.

Comfrey is the active ingredient in this ointment for bruises and sprains – it contains allantoin, which stimulates the growth of bone and soft tissue cells in the body. Comfrey can also be applied to the skin as a poultice.

INGREDIENTS
*200g/7oz petroleum jelly or paraffin wax
about 30g/1oz fresh comfrey leaves, roughly
chopped*

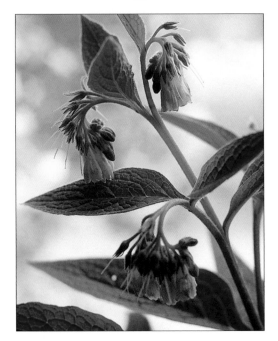

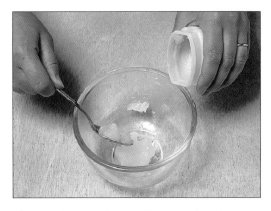

1 Put the petroleum jelly into a bowl.

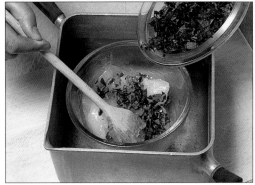

2 Set it set over a pan of boiling water, add the chopped comfrey leaves and stir well. Heat over gently simmering water for about 1 hour.

LEFT: An alternative country name for comfrey is "knitbone", a reference to its widespread use in healing wounds and speeding the recovery of fractures.

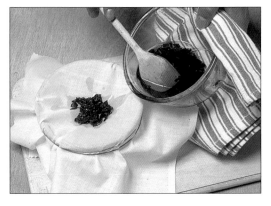

3 Strain the mixture through muslin secured to the rim of a jug with an elastic band. Pour immediately into a clean glass jar, before it has a chance to set.

> ### —VARIATIONS—
> Bruise ointments can also be made with houseleek (*Sempervivum tectorum*), yarrow (*Achillea millefolium*), or arnica flowers (*Arnica montana*). Follow the instructions for comfrey, substituting a similar quantity of plant material.

OPPOSITE: An ointment made with comfrey speeds the healing process for bruises and sprains.

> ### —CAUTION—
> In rare cases yarrow can cause an allergic reaction. Do not use arnica cream on broken skin as it may cause irritation.

LINIMENTS AND RUBS

A liniment is a liquid preparation, often made by mixing a herb oil with a tincture. Some liniments have an alcohol or vinegar base instead of oil.

Rheumatism Liniment

For rheumatic pains, aching joints and tired muscles, rub this liniment gently into the affected areas. It should be applied to the skin at body temperature.

INGREDIENTS
6 garlic cloves
300ml/1/2 pt/11/4 cups olive oil
30ml/2 tbsp tincture of juniper

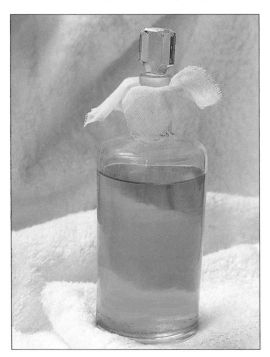

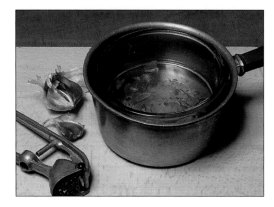

1 Crush the garlic cloves, without peeling them, and put them in a bowl. Pour the olive oil over the crushed garlic cloves. Cover the bowl with a piece of foil and stand it over a pan of simmering water. Heat gently for 1 hour. Check the water level in the pan regularly and top up as necessary.

2 Strain the oil, leave until lukewarm, then stir in the tincture of juniper and pour into a stoppered bottle. This liniment will keep for several months.

LEFT: The healing properties of garlic and juniper are harnessed to make a liniment for massaging aching joints and muscles.

RIGHT: Lavender and eucalyptus make a powerful combination for clearing a stuffy nose and are both strongly antiseptic.

OPPOSITE: A decongestant rub for colds and catarrh.

Lavender and Eucalyptus Vapour Rub for Colds

A blocked nose is a misery when suffering from a cold and prevents a sound night's sleep. This decongestant rub has a warming and soothing action and should be rubbed gently on to the throat, chest and back at bedtime, so that the vapours can be inhaled throughout the night. It can also be inhaled in boiling water.

INGREDIENTS
50g/2oz petroleum jelly
15ml/1 tbsp dried lavender
6 drops eucalyptus essential oil
4 drops camphor essential oil

1 Melt the petroleum jelly in a bowl over a pan of simmering water, stir in the lavender and heat for 30 minutes.

2 Strain the liquid jelly through muslin, leave to cool slightly, then add the essential oils. Pour into a clean jar and leave until set.

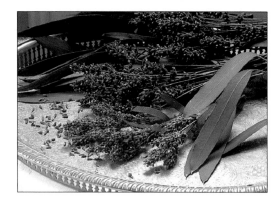

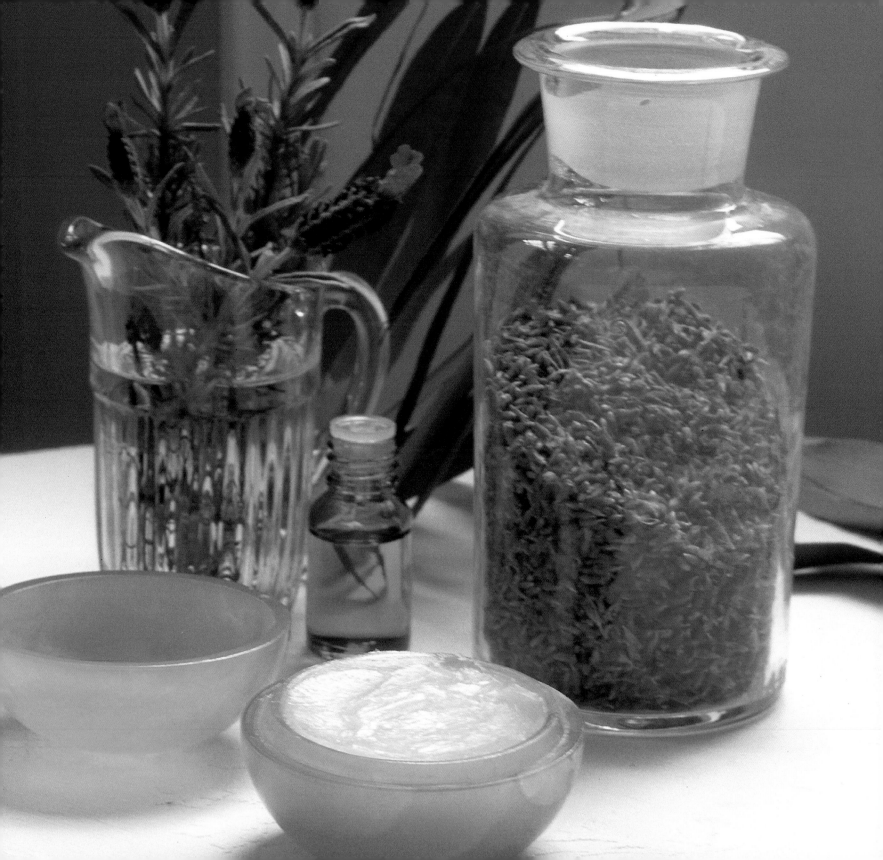

POULTICES

Healing poultices can be made from mashed herbs and other kitchen ingredients. Their purpose is to speed the healing of sprains, bruises and sores, to reduce inflammation or congestion, and to soothe abrasions. Always seek medical advice, however, if the condition does not clear up quickly.

Apply poultices directly to the skin or wrap in a clean piece of surgical gauze first. They may be used hot or cold: hot poultices are more effective for sprains and pains, while cold ones help to reduce heat if the area is inflamed.

Comfrey Poultice for Bruises and Sprains
Comfrey is effective as a treatment for bruises.

INGREDIENTS
handful of fresh comfrey leaves
boiling water

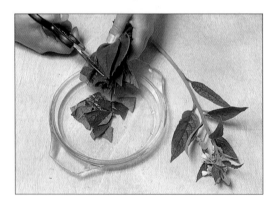

1 Snip a small handful of comfrey leaves into a dish. Cover the leaves with boiling water and mash to a thick pulp with a spoon.

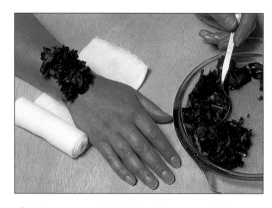

2 Leave to cool slightly, then spread the pulp directly on to the affected area. Cover lightly with a piece of gauze and bandage to hold the poultice in place. It should be left on for several hours.

BELOW: Fresh angelica leaves (top) with marjoram, was a favourite of the ancient Greeks for "hot fomentations".

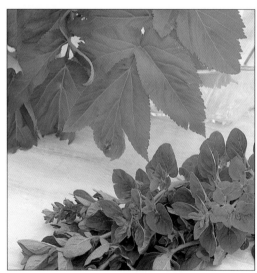

THERAPEUTIC POULTICES FOR OTHER COMMON PROBLEMS
ANGELICA AND MARJORAM POULTICE FOR ACHING JOINTS AND MUSCLES: Wild marjoram and angelica are both anti-inflammatory. Mix equal amounts of fresh or dried leaves and follow the method for Comfrey Poultice.
ANGELICA POULTICE FOR SUNBURN: Lightly crushed leaves and stems applied directly to the skin take the sting out of sunburn.
CARROT POULTICE FOR SORES AND CHAPPED SKIN: Carrots have good "drawing powers" for extracting toxins. Finely grate some fresh carrot and apply to the problem area.
SAGE POULTICE FOR GRAZES AND SCRAPES: Make a mash of the leaves, following the method for Comfrey Poultice, wrap it in a clean cloth and apply warm to the affected area.
OATMEAL POULTICE FOR STINGS AND BITES: Mix fine oatmeal to a paste with hot water or a herbal infusion – comfrey or marigold are the most suitable. Leave the paste until it is cold before applying to insect stings and bites.

OPPOSITE: A poultice is a quick and easy method of making use of the powers of the remarkable comfrey plant.

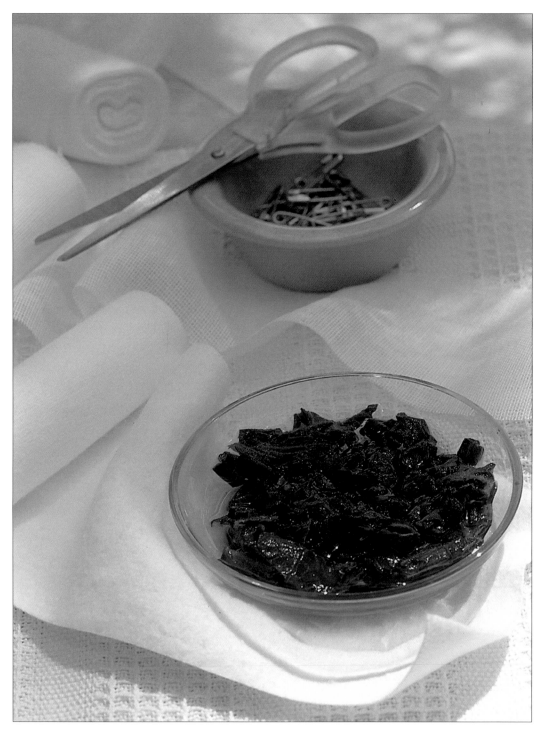

Slippery Elm and Thyme Poultice for Boils and Sores

The healing powers of slippery elm powder (made from the bark of the tree *Ulmus fulva*) are combined with the antiseptic properties of thyme to make a soothing poultice.

INGREDIENTS
small handful of thyme
boiling water
30ml/2 tbsp slippery elm powder

1 Strip the thyme leaves from the stalks (there should be about 15g/½ oz), put them on a saucer and cover with boiling water. Mash thoroughly and leave to cool.

2 Pour off some of the liquid, then add the slippery elm powder to make a coarse-textured paste. Apply directly to the skin or enclose in gauze first.

BELOW: Slippery elm powder with thyme.

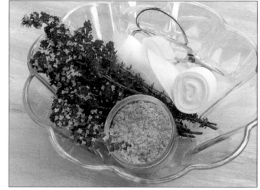

COMPRESSES

A cold compress will often alleviate a headache and a hot one helps soothe painful joints or strained muscles.

Lavender Compress for Headaches

Place a cool lavender compress across the forehead to relieve a tension headache. As soon as it gets warm, soak it again and re-apply.

INGREDIENTS
25g/1oz dried lavender
600ml/1 pint/2½ cups boiling water
3–4 drops lavender essential oil
10ml/2 tsp lavender tincture

1 To make the infusion, pour boiling water into a bowl over the dried lavender. Leave to stand for 1 hour, then strain. When cool, mix in the essential oil and tincture.

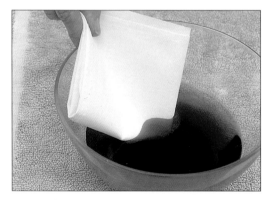

2 Fold a piece of soft cotton fabric into a loose pad. Soak it in the lavender infusion, and wring it out lightly.

—*HERBAL EYEPADS*—

A compress over eyes will refresh them, reduce puffiness, and relieve itchiness.
FENNEL: Make a decoction of fennel seeds by boiling 10ml/2 tsp seeds in 300ml/½ pint/1¼ cups purified water for 30 minutes. Strain and leave to cool, then use to soak cotton wool pads.
CHAMOMILE TEA-BAG: Use first to make chamomile tea then apply to the eyes when cool.
ROSEWATER: Soak cotton wool pads in an infusion of rose petals, made with purified water.

Valerian Compress for Swollen Joints

Make a decoction by simmering 25g/1oz of the dried root in 600ml/1pt/2½ cups water, in a covered pan, for 1 hour. Strain, soak a pad of soft cotton in the extract and apply hot.

Wormwood Compress for Bruises

Make an infusion, using 25g/1oz fresh wormwood, or 15g/½ oz dried, to 500ml/17fl oz/2¼ cups boiling water. Leave to stand for 30 minutes before straining. Apply when cool. It may also bring relief from insect bites.

BELOW: A lavender compress eases a headache.

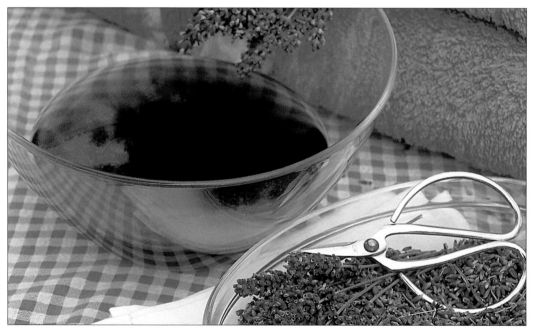

SINUS STEAM INHALANTS

Inhaling steam scented with aromatic herbs is an excellent way to relieve the congestion of a cold or blocked sinuses. There are several ways to do this.

Fresh Herb Inhalant

One of the simplest and most effective methods is to immerse freshly picked herbs and some spices in boiling water and breathe in the vapours. Choose from the following.

INGREDIENTS

HERBS: *eucalyptus leaves, basil, hyssop, juniper foliage, lavender, lemon balm, mint, rosemary, sage, thyme*
SPICES: *cayenne pepper, cinnamon stick, juniper berries*

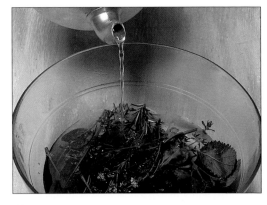

2 Pour in about 1 litre/1¾ pints/4 cups boiling water. Lean over the bowl, covering both it and your head with a towel.

Essential Oil Inhalant

INGREDIENTS

5 drops eucalyptus essential oil
2 drops camphor essential oil
1 drop citronella essential oil

Add the essential oils to 600ml/1 pint/2½ cups boiling water.

> —*DECONGESTANT ESSENTIAL OILS*—
> Cinnamon, eucalyptus, lavender, lemon, marjoram, peppermint, pine

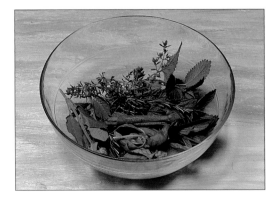

1 Put a large handful of selected herbs and spices in a bowl.

RIGHT: Inhaling the aromatic fragrance of freshly picked herbs is a simple and satisfying way to clear the nasal passages.

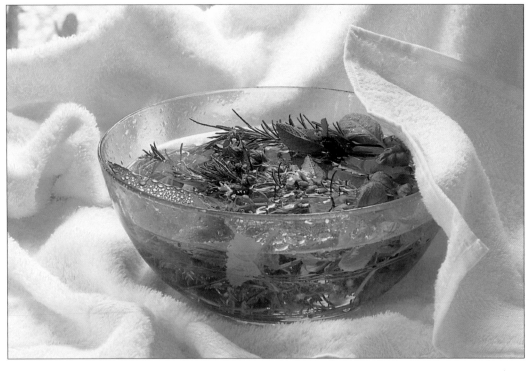

ESSENTIAL OIL BURNERS

Plant essential oils have a powerful effect on mood and mental states. Breathing in their vapours can be relaxing, restorative or uplifting. One way to inhale the scent is simply to put a few drops on a handkerchief and keep it on your pillow overnight. But for a more controlled and concentrated method, which is also longer lasting, an essential oil burner is the answer.

*BELOW: Jasmine (*Jasminum officinale*) has a relaxing, euphoric effect.*

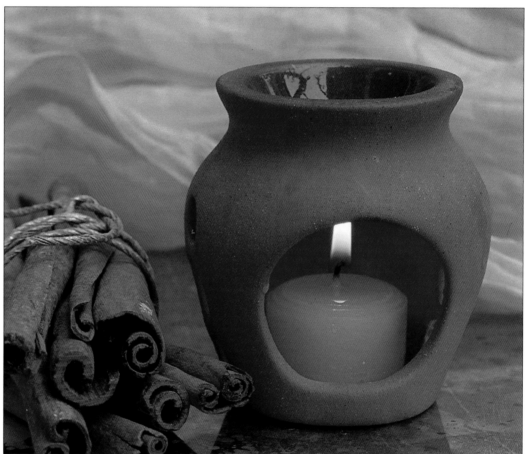

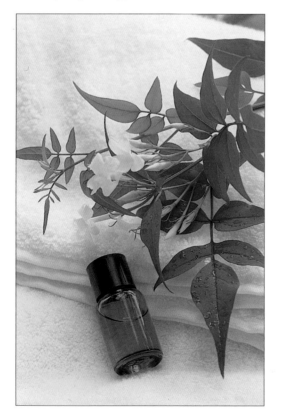

There is a wide range of styles to choose from, but they all work in a similar way by heating the essential oil in water so that it vaporizes as steam which can be inhaled. The heating element is usually a small candle or nightlight. Always treat an essential oil burner as you would a candle: do not leave it unattended or with an unsupervised child, and never leave one burning overnight.

ABOVE: A custom-made burner is the best way to inhale the therapeutic fragrance of plant essential oils.

Put 6–8 drops of essential oil into the filled water chamber of the burner. Top up the water as it evaporates, adding another 1–2 drops of oil as necessary. A few drops of oil in a bowl of hot water will also scent a room.

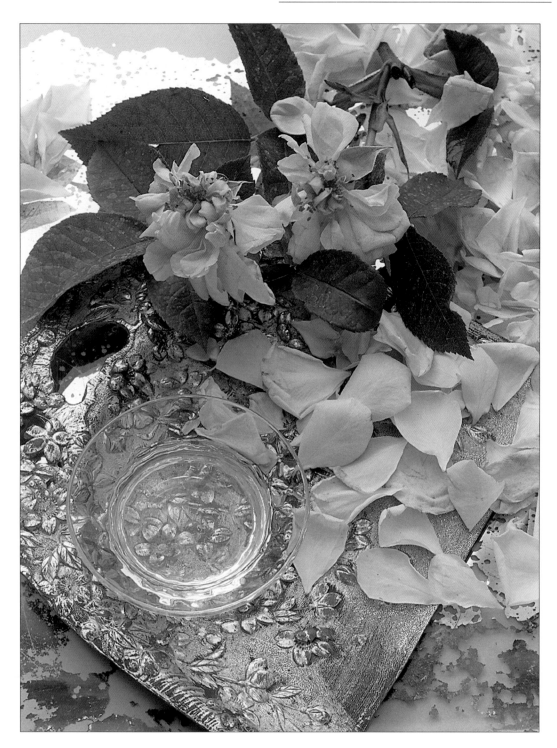

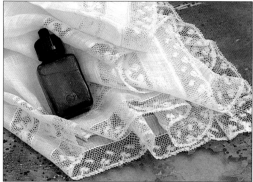

ABOVE: A drop or two on a handkerchief is a simple way to benefit from the aroma of essential oils.

LEFT: There can be few pleasanter ways of dealing with stress and anxiety than sitting back and breathing in the therapeutic fragrance of essential oils.

—ESSENTIAL OILS FOR THE NERVOUS SYSTEM—

RELAXING, RESTORATIVE OILS FOR DEPRESSION, NERVOUS TENSION, ANXIETY:

Basil, bergamot, camphor, chamomile, clary sage, frankincense, jasmine, lavender, neroli, rose, sandalwood, thyme, ylang-ylang.

SEDATIVE OILS FOR INSOMNIA:

Chamomile, juniper, lavender, marjoram, neroli, rose, sandalwood.

CALMING OILS FOR SHOCK AND STRESS:

Cedarwood, juniper, melissa, neroli, peppermint, rose.

STIMULATING OILS FOR APATHY, LETHARGY, MENTAL FATIGUE:

Basil, black pepper, cardamom, pennyroyal, peppermint, pine, rosemary.

SLEEP PILLOWS

Resting your head on a sleep pillow filled with mildly sedative herbs and flowers is very calming. Make a small cushion that you can tuck behind your neck or slip beneath your ordinary pillow. First make the sleep pot-pourri to go in the pillow.

Sleep Pot-pourri
INGREDIENTS
2 cups dried hop flowers
2 cups dried rose petals
1 cup dried chamomile flowers
1/2 cup each dried jasmine, orangeblossom and lavender
10ml/2 tsp ground orris root
5ml/1 tsp frankincense powder
5–6 drops neroli or melissa essential oil

Mix all the ingredients together, adding the essential oil last. Put into an airtight container and leave in a warm, dry place for at least 10 days, giving the container an occasional shake.

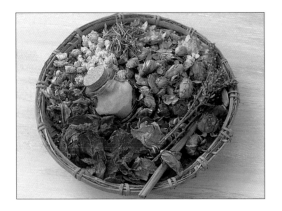

Sleep Pillow
YOU WILL NEED
cotton wadding (batting), 40 x 25cm/ 16 x 10in
pins and needles
sewing machine
matching sewing thread
sleep pot-pourri
2 pieces of fabric, 24 x 29cm/9 1/2 x 11 1/2 in
1m/1yd gathered broderie anglaise edging
tacking (basting) thread
22cm/8 1/2 in strip Velcro fastening

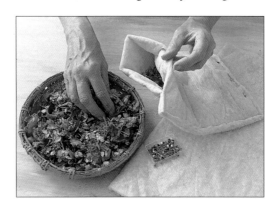

1 To make the inner pad, fold the cotton wadding (batting) in half with the shorter edges matching. Pin, then stitch the sides together, leaving an opening at one end. Turn through and fill the pillow with sleep pot-pourri. Slip-stitch the opening.

2 With the right side of one cover piece uppermost, and the broderie anglaise facing inwards, pin and tack (baste) the trim all around the edge.

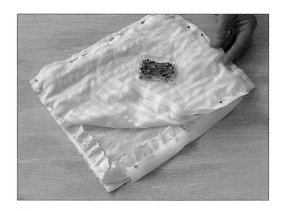

3 Separate the Velcro and stitch the two strips to matching short edges of the two cover pieces, with the right side of the fabric facing upwards. The Velcro should be centred. Pin the two cover pieces with right sides together, and stitch around the remaining three sides.

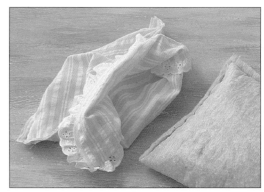

4 Turn the cover through and insert the filled pad. Fasten the Velcro.

FAR LEFT AND OPPOSITE: A sleep pillow filled with soothing herbs encourages a restful night.

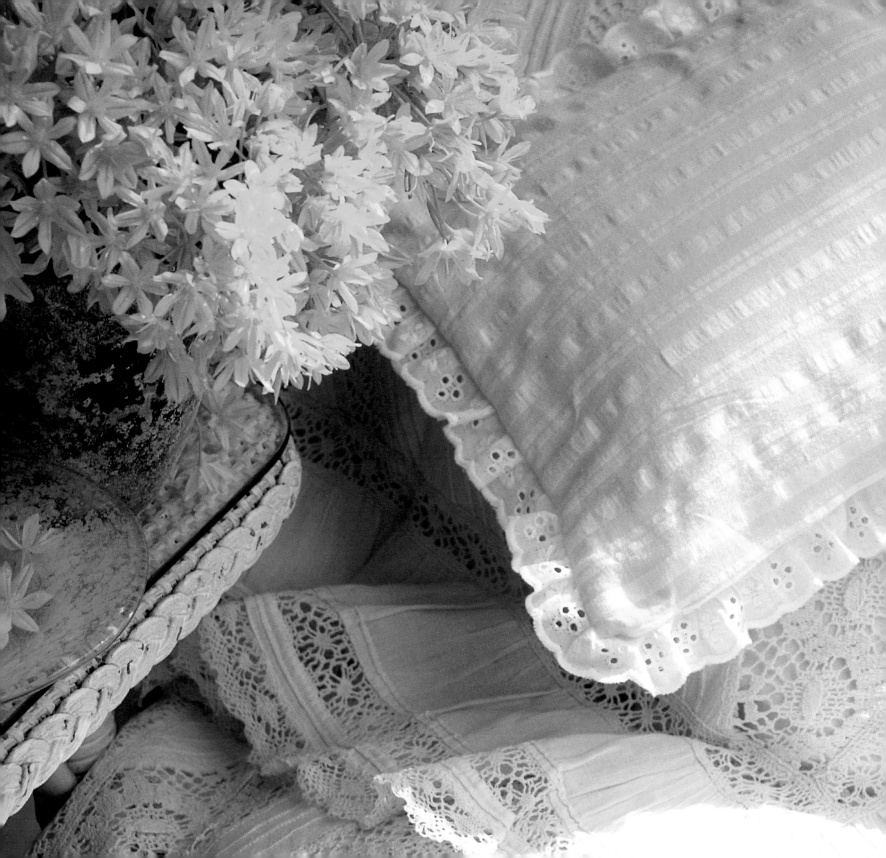

SWEET BAGS

Old herbals contain many recipes for aromatic powders to put into little bags to lay among linen or "wear in the pocket". While such sachets were used primarily for cosmetic purposes, they often had an equally important secondary purpose: to ward off infection or to deter moths, fleas and other pests and insects.

There is still a place for potent, but pleasant-smelling herbal sachets in drawers and cupboards to discourage moths. Filled with different pot-pourri mixtures, these little bags are pleasant to have around or to hang in the car to help alertness on journeys.

YOU WILL NEED
brown paper for pattern
scissors
pins
fine cotton or muslin fabric
pinking shears
pot-pourri filling
elastic bands
ribbon or tape

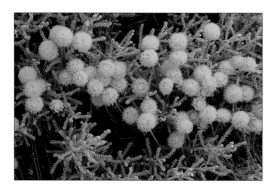

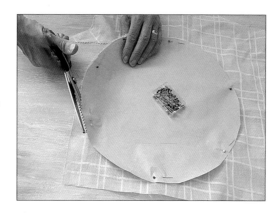

1 Cut out a circle of paper with a diameter of 30cm/12in – a dinner plate makes a useful template. Pin the paper pattern on to the fabric and cut around it with pinking shears.

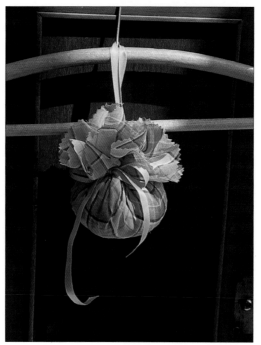

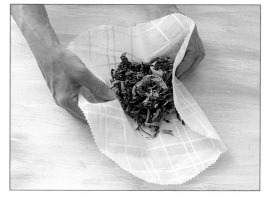

2 Fill the centre with enough pot-pourri to make a plump shape when gathered up.

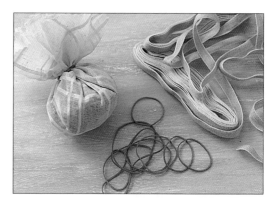

3 Gather up the fabric around the filling, fastening it at the neck with an elastic band. Tie the neck with ribbon or tape, and form a loop to hang up the bag.

FAR LEFT: Cotton lavender is strongly aromatic and dries well for use in pot-pourris.

LEFT: Hang an insect-repellent bag in the wardrobe to deter moths and pests.

—Sweet-bag Fillings—
Moth Bags

To deter moths from attacking your clothes and other bugs and beetles from the food cupboard, fill the sweet bags with insect-repellent herbs and spices and hang them in your wardrobe or kitchen.

Ingredients

DRIED HERBS: *bay, cotton lavender, lavender, pennyroyal, rosemary, southernwood, thyme, wormwood*
GROUND SPICES: *cinnamon, cloves ground orris root*
5–6 drops each lavender and clove essential oils
2 drops patchouli essential oil

Revival Bags

For a sachet to hang in the car, a pot-pourri mix based on rosemary and tangy citrus scents will help to maintain a clear and alert head.

Ingredients

DRIED HERBS: *lemon verbena, mint, rosemary, thyme*
dried orange and lemon peel
ground orris root
camphor essential oil
lemon essential oil

RIGHT: *Little bags filled with pot-pourri have many uses around the home.*

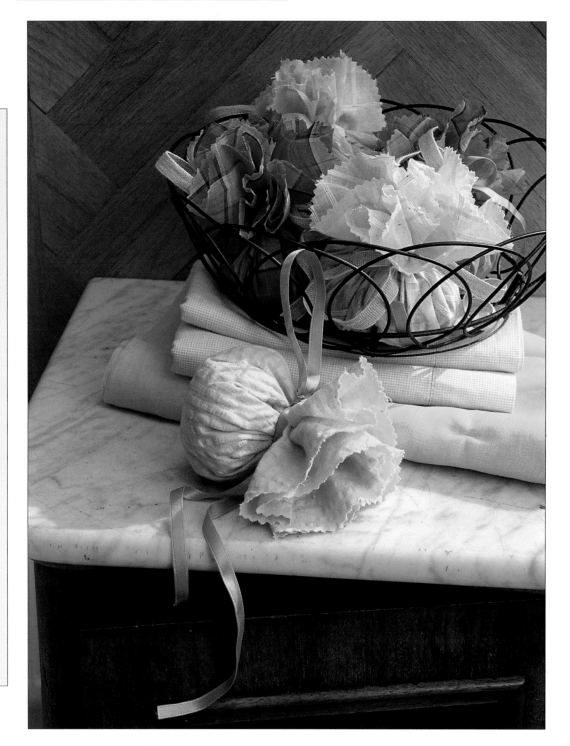

INSECT-REPELLENT LOTIONS

Many plants have insect-repellent properties. In India, neem leaves have been used for centuries against the onslaughts of moths and other insects, and in more northerly regions, the bog myrtle *(Myrica gale)* has proved an effective anti-midge shrub. Potent commercial pesticides for crops are made with pyrethrum *(Tanacetum cinerariifolium)* and derris *(Derris elliptica).*

Closer to home, we can make use of the properties of many common garden plants to make lotions to guard against midges and biting insects. Strong infusions of elder leaves, yarrow and wormwood make traditional anti-insect lotions and some people find feverfew tincture effective. The essential oils of lavender, lemon balm and citronella are also good standbys. Good quality, pure lavender oil can be applied undiluted to the skin; lemon balm and citronella should first be diluted in a vegetable carrier oil.

Yarrow and Elder Leaf Lotion

Collect a handful of fresh yarrow and two handfuls of elder leaves. Put them into a jug (pitcher), pour in 300ml/½ pint/1¼ cups boiling water and leave for 1 hour. Strain and pour into a bottle – a small atomizer bottle that you can carry with you is useful. Use within 2–3 days and discard any remainder.

RIGHT: If you do get bitten, rub a handful of basil or lemon balm leaves on to the skin.

Wormwood Lotion
INGREDIENTS
15g/½ oz dried wormwood
300ml/½ pint/1¼ cups boiling water
8 drops lavender essential oil or 15ml/1 tbsp lavender tincture
30ml/2 tbsp vodka

Put the wormwood into a jug and pour on the boiling water. Leave for 1 hour then strain and add the other ingredients. The alcohol helps to preserve this lotion, but keep it in a cool place.

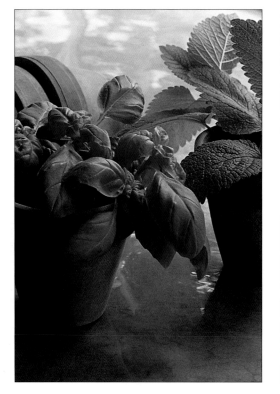

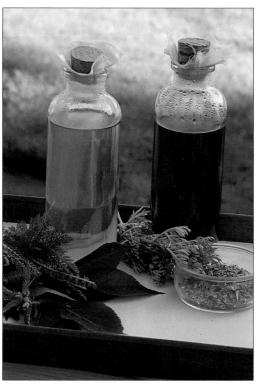

ABOVE: Herbs from the garden make useful insect-repellent lotions. (LEFT TO RIGHT): Yarrow and elder leaf lotion, wormwood lotion.

—*CAUTION*—
Remember herbs are powerful, so always try a small test patch on the skin if using a herbal infusion as an insect repellent for the first time, in case of allergies. Do not use insect-repellent lotions near the eyes. Do not use if pregnant or for children under five.

INSECT-REPELLENT CANDLES

It is not difficult to make your own candles. If you scent them with lavender or citronella essential oils they are a good way of deterring insects on summer evenings in the garden.

YOU WILL NEED
150g/5oz paraffin wax
15g/½ oz stearin
small and large saucepans
scissors
wick
candle mould
dowelling rod or pencil
mould sealant
wax colouring sticks
15–20 drops citronella or lavender essential oil

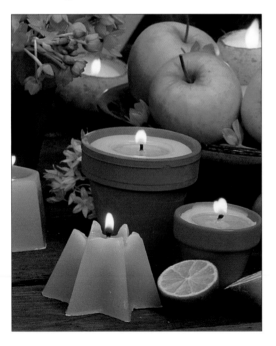

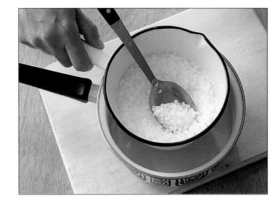

1 Over a large pan of boiling water, melt the paraffin wax and stearin in a small saucepan with a pouring lip.

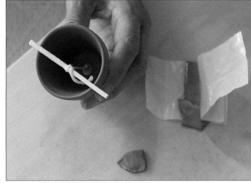

2 Cut a length of wick, about 5cm/2in longer than the height of the mould. Dip the wick in the melted wax, then thread it through the bottom of the mould and tie the end to a rod placed across the top. Pull the wick taut, and press sealant over the hole.

LEFT: Candles scented with essential oil deter insects when you are eating al fresco.

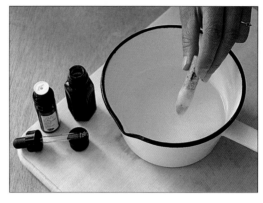

3 When the wax has melted, leave it over the heat for a further 2–3 minutes (it needs to reach a temperature of about 80°C/175°F). Dip in the wax colouring stick and stir to give the shade you require. Allow the wax to cool slightly before adding the citronella or lavender essential oil.

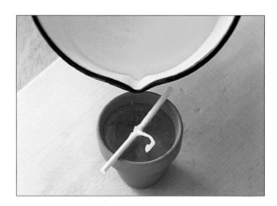

4 Pour the wax into the mould and allow it to settle, then tap the mould to free air bubbles. As the wax cools, a well will develop in the centre. Leave for about 2 hours to set, then pour more melted wax into the well.

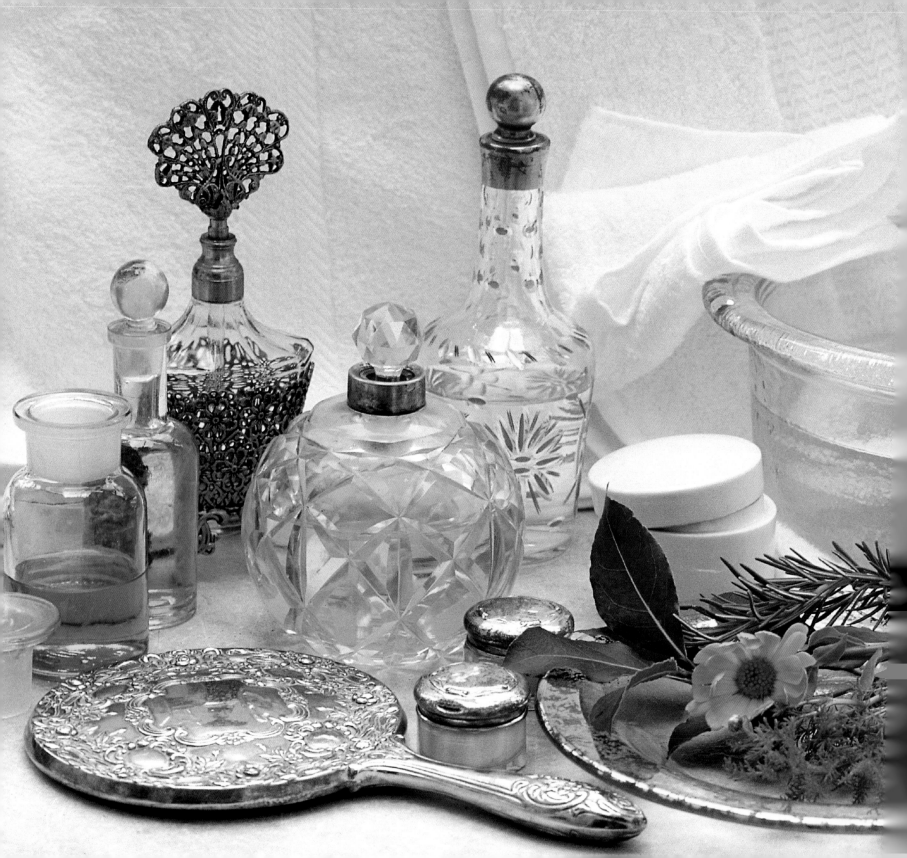

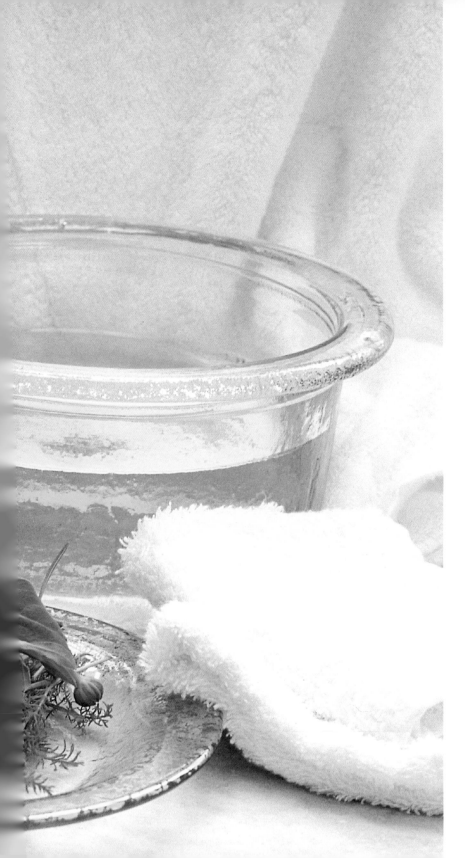

CHAPTER FOUR

HERBAL BEAUTY

———

"Take unto thee sweet spices, stacte, and onycha and galbanum – And thou shalt make it a perfume, a confection after the art of the apothecary."
EXODUS 30: 34–5

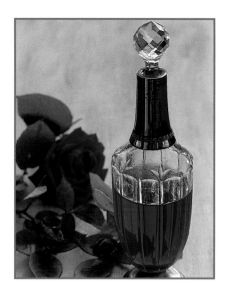

Many of the old herbals included advice on using herbs for beauty, and making perfumed preparations was part of the apothecary's art. Most of the recipes in this chapter are not solely cosmetic but are directed towards therapeutic beauty treatments and many have a secondary role in relieving minor ailments. All will promote general health through an enhanced sense of well-being.

ABOVE: Rose petals make a scented, soothing toner for the skin.

LEFT: Herbs and flowers provide the materials for simple beauty preparations.

BATH BAGS

In days gone by, baths were often taken as much for medicinal purposes as for hygiene. Gervase Markham, in *Countrey Contentments* (1623), gives recipes for several healing baths. He also includes "A generall bath for clearing the skin and comforting the body". He advises boiling herbs in milk then letting "the Party stand or sit in it an houre or two, and when they come out they must go to bed and beware of taking cold".

A rather simpler way of enjoying herbs in the bath is to put them into re-usable drawstring bags to hang from the tap while the water is running. This way, you avoid a messy residue of greenery in the plughole (drain).

A Drawstring Bath Bag
You can use any combination of pleasantly aromatic herbs, or choose from the list opposite to match a specific requirement.

YOU WILL NEED
25cm/10in square of calico or fine cotton fabric
ruler
tailor's chalk
sewing machine
matching sewing thread
70cm/28in tape
safety pin or bodkin
pins

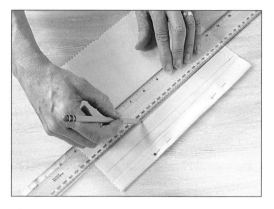

1 Turn over the top of the fabric to a depth of 6cm/2½ in to form a hem. Mark a line 3cm/1¼ in from the folded edge. Stitch along this line and along the hem edge.

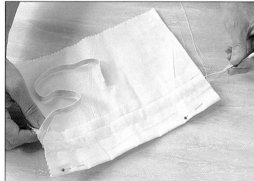

2 Feed the tape through the channel formed by the lines of stitching. Fold the fabric in half, right sides together. Stitch the edges, leaving the channel open.

LEFT: *To soften hard water, add 15ml/1 tbsp fine oatmeal to the bag. You could also add a piece of soap and use as a herbal scrub.*

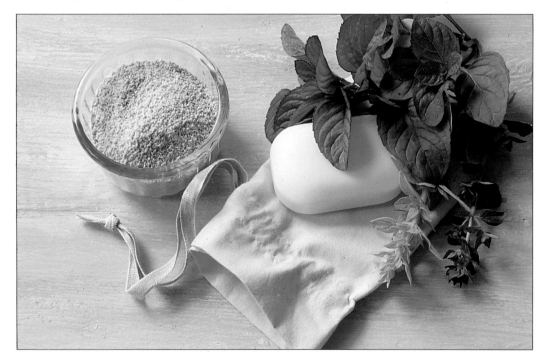

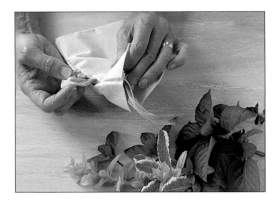

3 Turn the bag to the right side. Fill with a handful of mixed fresh herbs and pull the neck tight.

RIGHT: For a restorative invigorating bath, hang a herb-filled bath bag over the tap while the water is running, then stir 1kg/2¼ lb sea salt into the bath. Soak in it for 10 minutes before scrubbing the skin with the bath bag, to which you have added some grated soap. Finish with a cool shower.

—HERBAL BATH MIXES—

RELAXING: Chamomile flowers and foliage.
REVITALIZING: Rosemary, peppermint, lemon thyme, pine needles.
TO IMPROVE CIRCULATION: Nettles. These will lose their sting once they have been soaked in hot water.
FOR ACHES AND PAINS: Comfrey leaves with 15ml/1 tbsp powdered ginger.
FOR COLDS: Lavender, thyme and a 2.5cm/1in piece of grated fresh ginger.
FOR ITCHY SKIN: Comfrey, houseleek, lady's mantle, marshmallow. Add a cup of cider vinegar to the bath as well.

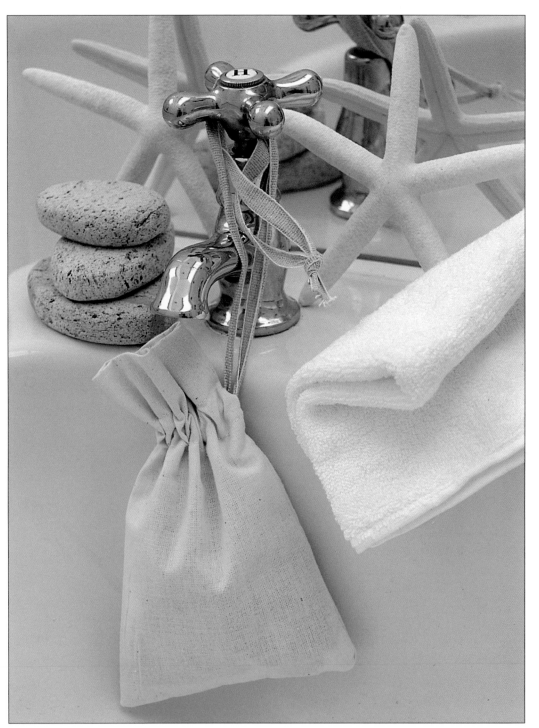

BATH OILS AND LOTIONS

Herbal baths can be used for a range of therapeutic purposes, as well as to relax the mind and body. Instead of adding fresh herbs in bath bags, plant essential oils can be added directly to the water. Measure essential oil straight from the bottle, squeezing about 5 drops into a full bath. Do not add the oil while the water is still running as it will evaporate too quickly and be wasted.

Milk and Honey Bath Oil with Rosemary

Milk is well known for its cleansing and lubricating qualities when applied to the skin. The addition of a little shampoo makes this a dispersing oil which does not leave a greasy rim around the bath.

INGREDIENTS
2 eggs
45ml/3 tbsp rosemary herb oil
10ml/2 tsp honey
10ml/2 tsp baby shampoo
15ml/1 tbsp vodka
150ml/¹⁄4 pint/²⁄3 cup milk

Beat the eggs and oil together, then add the other ingredients and mix thoroughly. Pour into a clean glass bottle. Add 30–45ml/2–3 tbsp to the bath and keep the rest chilled, for use within a few days.

RIGHT: A bath lotion made with honey and rosemary oil leaves skin smooth and silky.

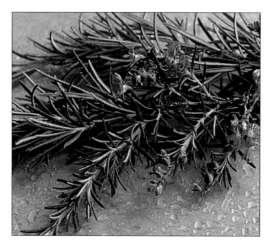

ABOVE: Rosemary has an invigorating scent and is rich in essential oil.

---**THERAPEUTIC BATH OILS**---

Mix two or three essential oils together in a base of sweet almond oil or jojoba oil. The quantities given are for a 50ml/¹⁄4 cup bottle of base oil. Add 20 drops of the mixed oil to the bath.

ANTI-STRESS MIX: 10 drops each marjoram, lavender and sandalwood.

INVIGORATING MIX: 5 drops rosemary, 5 drops camphor, 20 drops peppermint.

FOR COLDS AND FLU: 10 drops each eucalyptus, thyme and lavender.

FOR ARTHRITIS: 30 drops eucalyptus.

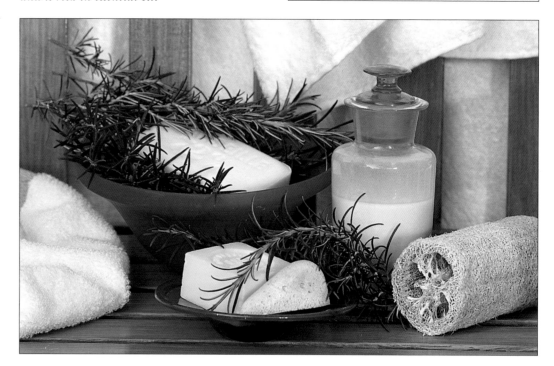

Coconut and Orangeflower Body Lotion

This creamy preparation is wonderfully nourishing for dry skin. Wheatgerm oil is rich in vitamin E, an antioxidant which protects skin cells against premature ageing.

INGREDIENTS
50g/2 oz coconut oil
60ml/4 tbsp sunflower oil
10ml/2 tsp wheatgerm oil
10 drops orangeflower essence or 5 drops neroli essential oil

1 Melt the coconut oil in a bowl over gently simmering water. Stir in the sunflower and wheatgerm oils.

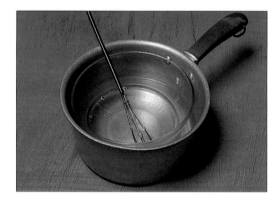

2 Leave to cool, then add the fragrance and pour into a jar. The lotion will solidify after several hours.

RIGHT: Coconut and orangeflower lotion is nourishing for the skin.

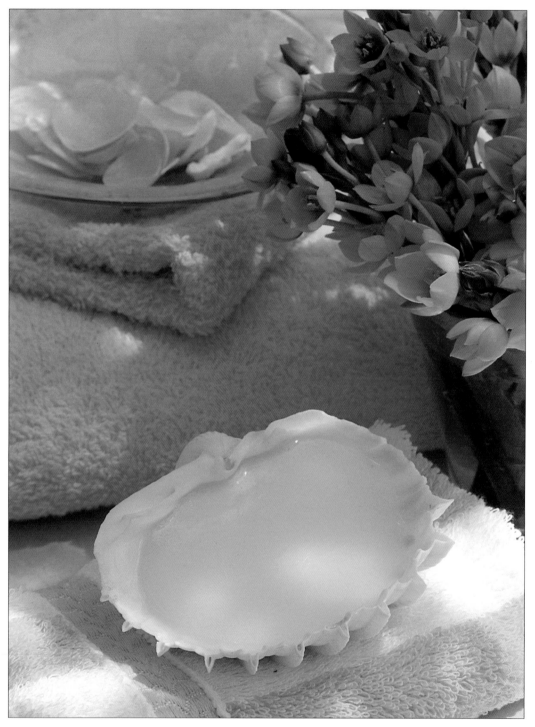

CHAMOMILE STEAM FACIAL

An occasional facial steam treatment deep-cleans the skin. The heat relaxes the pores and boosts blood circulation. With the addition of herbs, the stimulating and cleansing action of the steam is increased. Always close the pores afterwards by dabbing with a cooled skin toner appropriate to your skin type or by using a face mask. Steam facials should be avoided altogether by those with a tendency to thread veins.

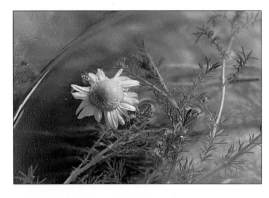

LEFT: Chamomile has a gentle, cleansing action, which suits most skin types, and a fresh apple scent.

BELOW: A steam treatment relaxes and softens the skin. Make it with an infusion of dried herbs, or simply float fresh herbs in boiling water.

INGREDIENTS

40g/1½ oz fresh or 15g/½ oz dried chamomile flowers
600ml/1 pint/2½ cups boiling water

Make a strong infusion of the fresh or dried flowers in boiling water. Leave to stand for 30 minutes, then strain. Re-heat the infusion, pour it into a bowl and, keeping your face about 30cm/12in above the steam, cover both head and basin with a towel for about 30 seconds. Repeat two or three times.

—VARIATION—

For a quick method, instead of making an infusion, float fresh chamomile flowers and leaves in hot water. You could also use mint, marjoram, marigolds or rose petals. Or, for extra fragrance, try adding a few drops of an essential oil such as lavender to the water.

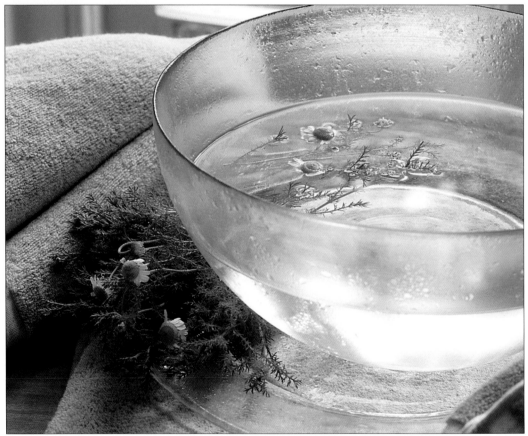

FACE MASKS

Herbal face masks tighten the skin, leaving it smooth and fresh. They help to heal blemishes, refine open pores, nourish and soothe. It is best not to use them too often as they can be over-stimulating.

RIGHT: Oatmeal helps remove grime, wheatgerm oil, honey and egg yolk are nourishing for dry skin.

BELOW: Oily skins benefit from the astringency of sage, parsley and lemon juice.

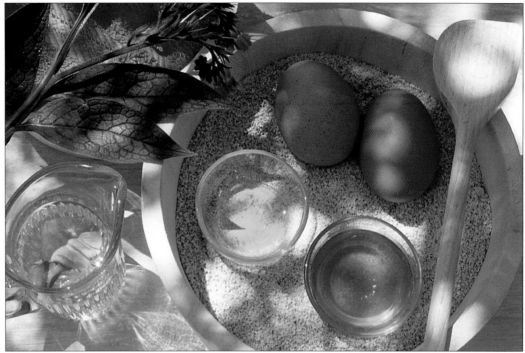

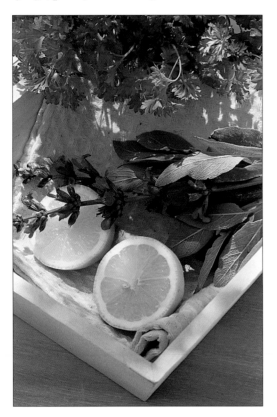

Comfrey and Rosewater Mask

This mask is ideal for nourishing dry skin.

INGREDIENTS
6 comfrey leaves
150ml/¼ pint/⅔ cup boiling water
30ml/2 tbsp fine oatmeal
1 egg yolk
5ml/1 tsp honey
5ml/1 tsp rosewater
5 drops wheatgerm oil
a little milk or yogurt to mix

Infuse the comfrey leaves in boiling water and leave until cool before straining. Mix 15ml/1 tbsp of this infusion with the other ingredients to make a smooth paste. Apply evenly to the face, avoiding the eye area. Leave for 10–15 minutes then rinse off.

Parsley and Sage Mask for Oily Skin

This formula has a drying effect on the skin and should not be over-used.

INGREDIENTS
15g/½ oz fresh parsley
15g/½ oz fresh sage
300ml/½ pint/1¼ cups boiling water
30ml/2 tbsp fine oatmeal
15ml/1 tbsp fuller's earth
1 egg white
5ml/1 tsp lemon juice

Infuse the parsley and sage in the boiling water and leave to cool before straining. Mix 30–45ml/2–3 tbsp of the infusion with the other ingredients to make a smooth paste. Leave on the face for 15 minutes.

SKIN TONERS

Infusions of flowers and herbs make excellent skin toners. Apply with cotton wool (cotton balls) after removing a face mask or make-up, or use at any time to freshen the skin. These toners must be kept chilled and used up within a few days as they soon deteriorate.

Rose Petal Toner for Sensitive Skin

Any fragrant roses are suitable for this recipe, as long as they have not been sprayed with pesticide. Pink or red ones are best.

INGREDIENTS
40g/1½ oz fresh rose petals
600ml/1 pint/2½ cups boiling water
15ml/1 tbsp cider vinegar

Put the rose petals in a bowl, pour over the boiling water and add the vinegar. Cover and leave to stand for 2 hours, then strain into a clean bottle.

RIGHT: *Dark red roses are best for colour. The toner on the left is made from fragrant 'Ena Harkness', with elderflower on the right.*

—*VARIATION*—
Elderflower Toner for Dry Skin
INGREDIENTS
25g/1oz dried elderflowers
600ml/1 pint/2½ cups boiling water

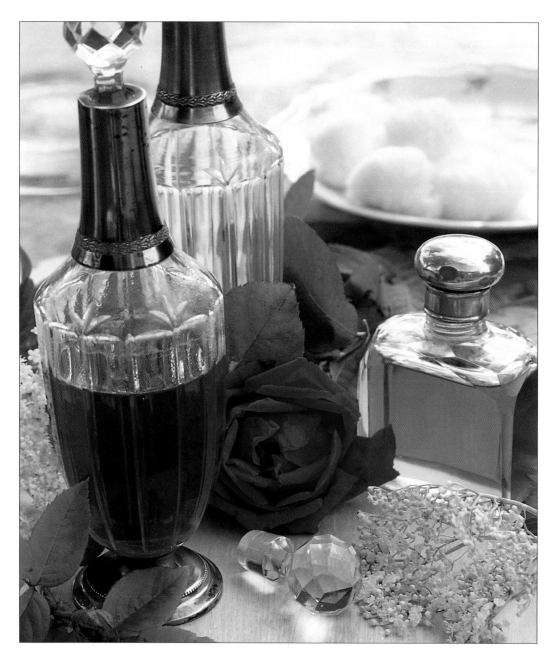

Marigold Milk for Inflamed Skin and Thread Veins

Pot marigold flowers are soothing and healing. Thread veins are not going to disappear if you use this preparation, but its cooling action does help. Remember that sun, extremes of temperature and too much alcohol all make the condition worse. The calendula oil used here is an infused vegetable oil, not an essential oil.

INGREDIENTS
6–8 fresh pot marigold flowers
300ml/1/2 pint/1 1/4 cups milk
3 drops tincture of benzoin
5ml/1 tsp calendula oil

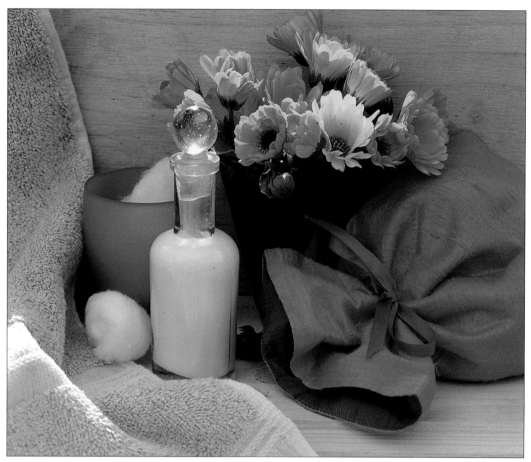

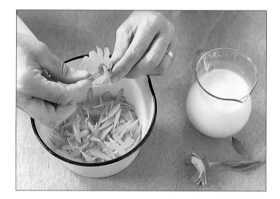

1 Pull the petals off the marigold flowerheads and put them in an enamel pan. Pour in the milk, cover and simmer gently for about 30 minutes.

2 Remove from the heat and stir in the tincture of benzoin and calendula oil. Leave until cool, then strain into a jug (pitcher).

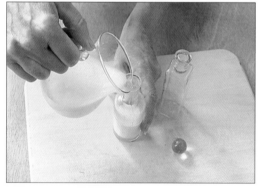

3 Pour the marigold milk into a glass bottle. Keep the lotion chilled and use within 3 days to soothe the skin.

ABOVE: *Apply soothing marigold milk to the face with cotton wool (cotton balls).*

—VARIATION—
Mint and Marigold Toner for Oily Skin
INGREDIENTS
25g/1oz fresh mint leaves
15g/1/2 oz fresh pot marigold petals
600ml/1 pint/2 1/2 cups boiling water
30ml/2 tbsp vodka

ELDERFLOWER MOISTURIZER

Amoisturizing cream is a must to prevent dryness, keep wrinkles at bay and protect from wind and weather. Making your own ensures the use of simple ingredients and herbs that will be gentle on your skin. This recipe includes elderflowers which have a long-standing reputation for lightening the skin.

INGREDIENTS
15g/¹/₂ oz dried elderflowers
600ml/1 pint/2¹/₂ cups boiling water
30ml/2 tbsp emulsifying ointment
5ml/1 tsp beeswax
30ml/2 tbsp almond oil
2.5ml/¹/₂ tsp borax

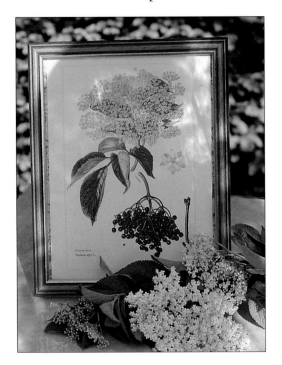

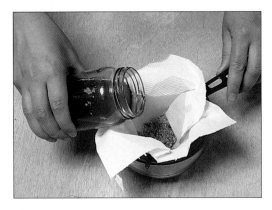

1 Make the elderflower infusion by pouring the boiling water over the dried elderflowers in a jar. Leave to stand for 30 minutes, then strain. You will need 120ml/4floz/¹/₂ cup for this recipe. Keep the remainder, chilled, to use as a skin toner.

LEFT: The Anatomie of the Elder (1644) devoted 230 pages to detailing the virtues of the plant. "Medicinal in every part", it was made into every form of remedy from syrups, tinctures and conserves to liniments, vinegars, decoctions, baths and powders.

OPPOSITE: Elderflowers add their unique therapeutic properties to this light-textured moisturizing cream.

—— *VARIATIONS* ——
Other herbs, such as comfrey or pot marigolds, can be substituted for elderflowers.

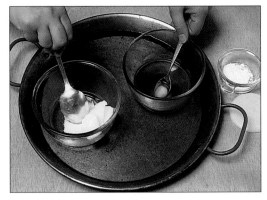

2 Put the emulsifying ointment, beeswax and almond oil into one bowl, and the elderflower infusion and borax into another. Set them both over hot water and stir until the oils are melted and the borax is dissolved. Borax helps to bind the ingredients.

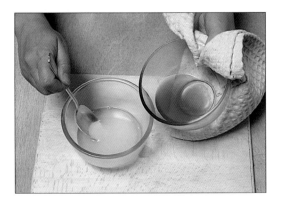

3 Remove from the heat and pour the elderflower mixture into the oils, beating gently until incorporated. Leave to cool, stirring at intervals. Pour the cream into a jar before it sets completely. It will keep for several months.

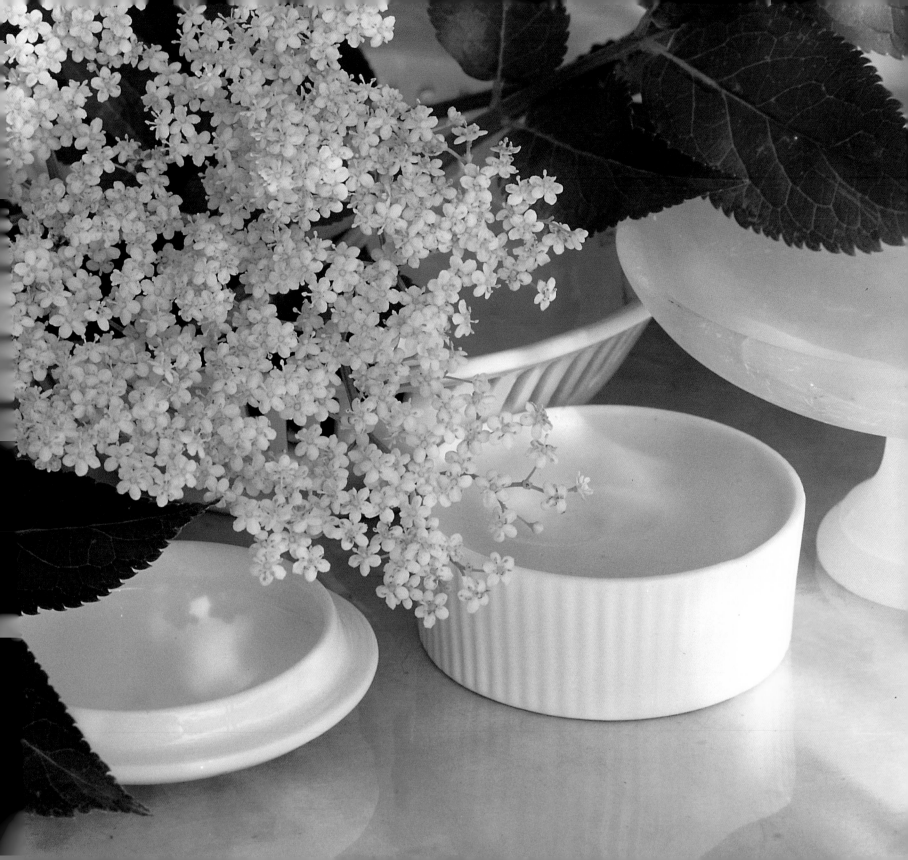

HERBAL SHAMPOO

The easiest way to make a herbal shampoo is to add 30–45ml/2–3 tbsp of a strong herbal infusion to a mild baby shampoo. Alternatively, you could add 2–3 drops of your favourite essential oil. However, the traditional herb for cleansing the hair is soapwort.

Soapwort Shampoo

If you are used to a detergent-based shampoo, you will find this does not lather in the same way, although it will froth up if you whisk it. The gentle cleansing properties of soapwort shampoo are very beneficial if you suffer from an itchy scalp or dandruff.

INGREDIENTS
25g/1oz fresh soapwort root, leaves and stem or
15g/1/2 oz dried soapwort root
750ml/1¼ pints/3 cups water
lavender water or eau-de-Cologne

Break up the soapwort stems, roughly chop the root and put the whole lot into a pan with the water. Bring to the boil and simmer for 20 minutes. Strain off the herbs and add a dash of lavender water or eau-de-Cologne, as soapwort does not have a very pleasant scent. Use like an ordinary shampoo, rubbing well into the scalp and rinsing.

— CAUTION —
Soapwort should never be taken
internally as it can be mildly poisonous.

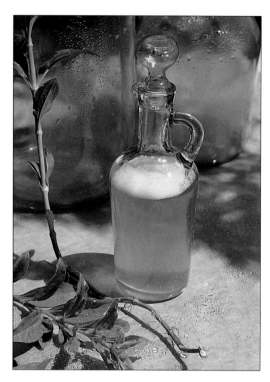

ABOVE: The cleansing properties of soapwort (Saponaria officinalis) are due to the saponins it contains. If you do not have access to the fresh plant, use the dried root instead.

Pure Soap Shampoo

All commercial shampoos contain some form of detergent, which is inclined to strip the hair of its natural oils. Pure soap is kinder, but it can leave hair dry and dulled. Rinse well with water, followed by a herbal rinse. Keep a jar of shampoo base, made by dissolving 115g/4oz pure soap flakes in 1 litre/1¾ pints/4 cups spring water, adding herbs as required.

Chamomile and Orangeflower Shampoo
INGREDIENTS
60ml/4 tbsp shampoo base
15ml/1 tbsp chamomile infusion
5 drops neroli essential oil

Mix the chamomile infusion and essential oil into the shampoo base just before washing your hair.

BELOW: A shampoo base, made with pure soap flakes, will keep indefinitely. Add a chamomile infusion or essential oils each time you use it.

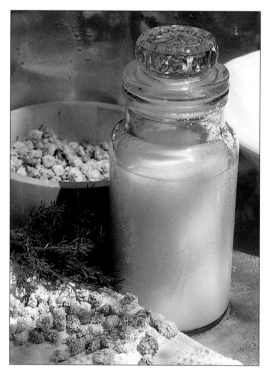

HERBAL HAIR RINSES

A herbal rinse helps to keep the hair shiny and in good condition. Make one up fresh before you start to wash your hair. Hold your head over a portable bowl as you pour the herbal rinse through your hair. Keep pouring the rinse from the bowl back into the jug (pitcher) and re-apply at least six times.

Chamomile Rinse for Fair Hair

INGREDIENTS

25g/1 oz dried chamomile flowers or 40g/1 ½ oz fresh flowers and leaves

1 litre/1¾ pints/4 cups boiling water

Put the flowers into a jug (pitcher), pour in the boiling water and leave to stand for 1 hour. Strain off the herbs through a sieve lined with kitchen paper (paper towel).

Rosemary Rinse for Dark Hair

Rosemary has a high essential oil content and is also beneficial for dry hair.

INGREDIENTS

40g/1½ oz fresh rosemary

1 litre/1¾ pints/4 cups boiling water

Make in the same way as the Chamomile Rinse. Use frequently for shiny hair.

RIGHT: To gain maximum benefit from a herbal rinse, catch it in a bowl and re-apply.

Nettle Rinse for Dandruff

INGREDIENTS

25g/1oz nettle leaves

25g/1oz nasturtium flowers and leaves

1 litre/1¾ pints/4 cups water

30ml/2 tbsp cider vinegar

30ml/2 tbsp witch hazel

Boil the water and pour it over the nettles and nasturtiums. Nettles loose their sting in boiling water. Leave to stand overnight, then strain off the herbs and add the vinegar and witch hazel. Pour through the hair as a final rinse every time you shampoo.

A Lotion for Dandruff and Dry, Itching Scalp

INGREDIENTS

115g/4oz mixed fresh herbs: lavender, nasturtium, nettle, pot marigold, rosemary, southernwood, thyme

1 litre/1¾ pints/4 cups water

120ml/4fl oz/½ cup vodka

Put the herbs into a large enamel pan with the water and simmer gently for 40 minutes. Leave for eight hours. Strain and add the vodka. Apply liberally to the scalp on cotton wool 2–3 times a week.

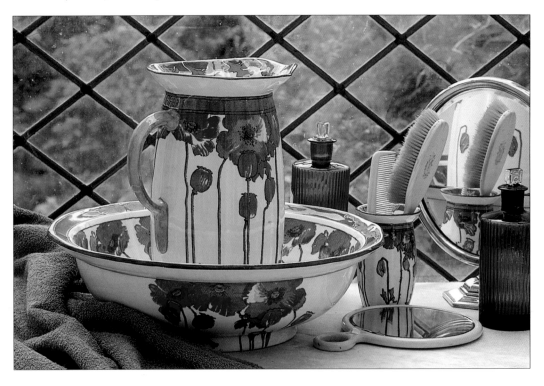

HAND TREATMENTS

Gardening, domestic chores and the demands of daily living can all take their toll on hands. Use garden roses to redress the balance.

Rose Infusion

Make this rose infusion before making the mask.

INGREDIENTS
large handful of fragrant rose petals
600ml/1pint/2½ cups boiling water
30ml/2 tbsp vodka

Put the rose petals into a bowl and pour in the boiling water. Leave to stand for 30 minutes, then add the vodka and strain off the petals.

Rose Hand Mask

This is a good way to restore the tone and texture of the skin – and also forces you to relax for 15 minutes. Smooth on the Rose Hand Lotion afterwards.

INGREDIENTS
45ml/3 tbsp medium or fine oatmeal
30ml/2 tbsp rose infusion or triple-distilled rosewater
5ml/1 tsp almond oil
5ml/1 tsp lemon juice
5ml/1 tsp glycerine

BELOW: *Roses 'Ena Harkness'* (LEFT) *and 'Zéphirine Drouhin' are strongly perfumed.*

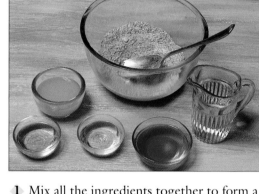

1 Mix all the ingredients together to form a soft paste. You may need to add a little extra rose infusion if it seems too stiff.

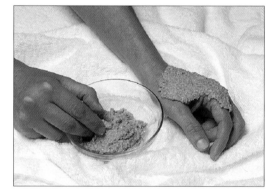

2 Take yourself to a quiet room where you aren't going to be interrupted, then spread the mask all over the backs of the hands and the fingers. Leave it in place for 15 minutes.

3 Rinse off the hand mask in warm water to leave hands feeling soft and smooth. Follow the treatment with a liberal application of Rose Hand Lotion.

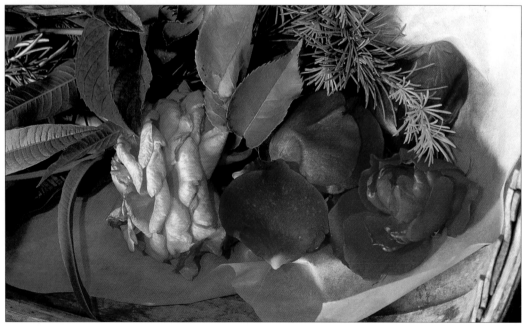

Rose Hand Lotion

This recipe is best made in small quantities so that you can use it fresh, ideally within a week. Although it feels sticky when you first apply it, it soon disappears, leaving hands silky. Shake well before each application.

INGREDIENTS
90ml/6 tbsp glycerine
30ml/2 tbsp rose infusion
10ml/2 tsp triple-distilled rosewater
10ml/2 tsp cornflour

Mix the glycerine, rose infusion and rosewater together, then add the cornflour and beat until it is incorporated.

RIGHT: *A lotion of rosewater and glycerine keeps hands smooth.*

BELOW: *Make a rose infusion by pouring boiling water over fragrant petals.*

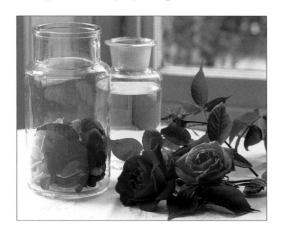

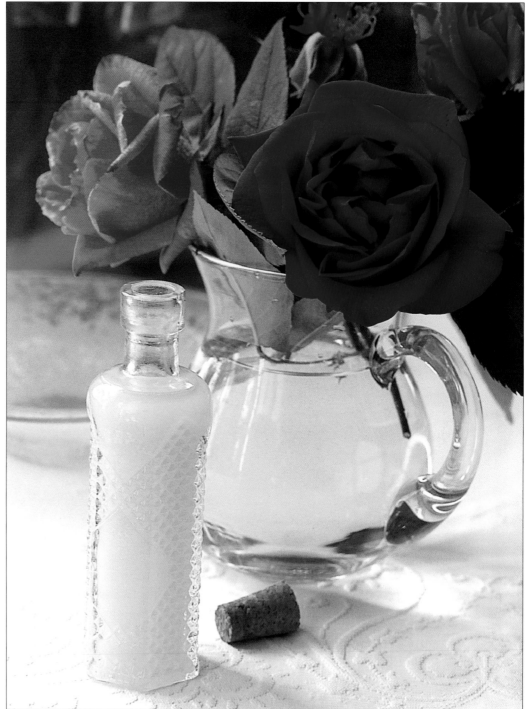

HERBAL FOOT BATHS

There is nothing like a fragrant foot bath for refreshing tired feet. At the same time, it revitalizes the whole being, its warmth relaxes the body and the scent of the herbs calms the mind. Foot baths are also comforting if you have a cold and, with the right herbs, they can help fight fungal infection.

RIGHT: Make a strong infusion and add it to a basin of water.

BELOW: Fresh herbs, collected from the garden, make a restorative foot bath for aching feet.

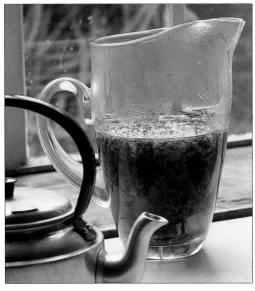

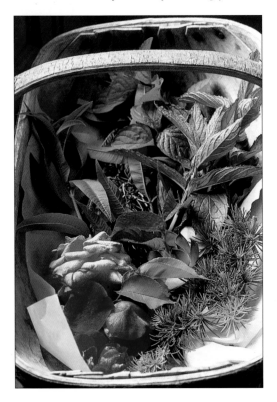

Herbal Foot Bath for Aching Feet
INGREDIENTS
50g/2oz mixed fresh herbs: peppermint, yarrow, pine needles, chamomile flowers, rosemary, houseleek
1 litre/1¾ pints/4 cups boiling water
15ml/1 tbsp borax
15ml/1 tbsp Epsom salts

Roughly chop the herbs, put them in a large bowl and pour in the boiling water. Leave to stand for 1 hour. Strain, and add to a basin containing about 1.75 litres/3 pints/7½ cups hot water – the final temperature of the foot bath should be comfortably warm. Stir in the borax and Epsom salts. Immerse the feet and soak for 15–20 minutes.

Antifungal Foot Bath
This foot bath is suitable for athlete's foot. The cider vinegar helps to restore the pH balance of the skin, which becomes over-alkaline when suffering from this condition. Myrrh and tea tree oil both have antifungal properties.

INGREDIENTS
25g/1oz dried sage
25g/1oz dried pot marigold flowers
1 large aloe vera leaf, chopped
15ml/1 tbsp myrrh granules
2.2 litres/4 pints/9 cups water
10 drops tea tree essential oil
60ml/4 tbsp cider vinegar

Simmer the herbs and myrrh in the water for 20 minutes. Leave to cool a little, then strain and add the tea tree oil and the cider vinegar. Immerse the feet for 15 minutes. Dry them thoroughly afterwards.

Lemon Verbena and Lavender Foot Bath
INGREDIENTS
15g/½ oz dried lemon verbena
30ml/2 tbsp dried lavender
5 drops lavender essential oil
30ml/2 tbsp cider vinegar

Put the lemon verbena and lavender in a basin and pour in enough hot water to cover the feet. When it has cooled add the lavender oil and cider vinegar.

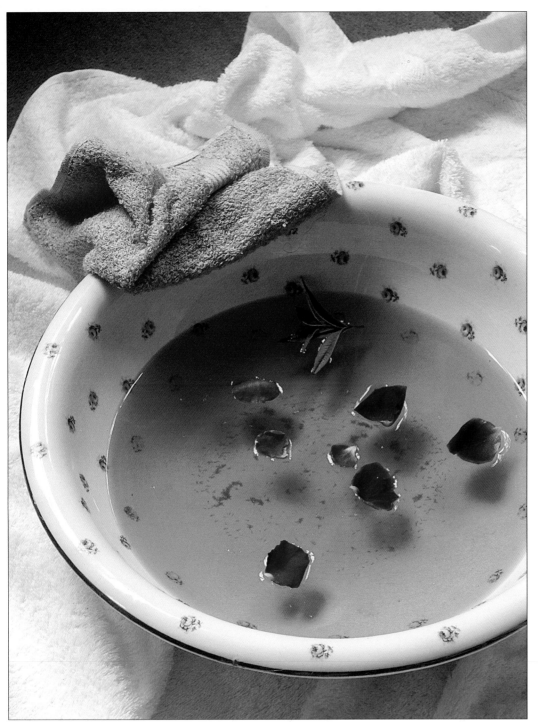

Mustard Foot Bath

This has long been a popular treatment for colds and chills. It has a warming effect and is extremely comforting.

INGREDIENTS
15ml/1 tbsp mustard powder
2.2 litres/4 pints/9 cups hot water

Stir the mustard into the water until it is dissolved. Immerse the feet while the bath is still hot. Re-heat if required.

LEFT: A foot bath restores and revitalizes the whole body.

BELOW: A mustard foot bath is a popular treatment for relieving colds and chills that has stood the test of time.

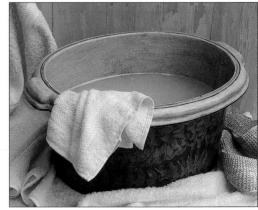

MOUTHWASHES AND TOOTH POWDERS

Herbs can be used in many ways to keep breath fresh and teeth clean. Gervase Markham in *Countrey Contentments* (1623) includes directions for pounding sage and salt into a powder "for teeth that are yellow".

Sage and Salt Tooth Powder
INGREDIENTS
25g/1oz fresh sage leaves
60ml/4 tbsp sea salt

BELOW: *A combination of sage and salt is traditionally used for cleaning the teeth.*

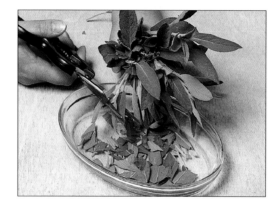

1 With a pair of scissors, shred the sage leaves into an ovenproof dish.

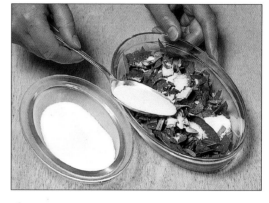

2 Mix in the salt, grinding it into the leaves with a wooden spoon or pestle. Bake the mixture in a very low oven for about 1 hour, until dry and crisp.

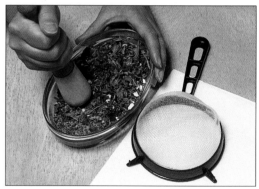

3 Pound it down again until reduced to a powder. Use on a damp toothbrush instead of toothpaste.

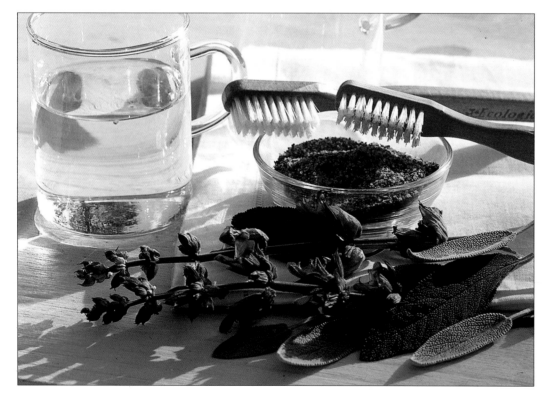

—*VARIATIONS*—
For a milder effect, substitute 1 tablespoon of orris root powder for salt.

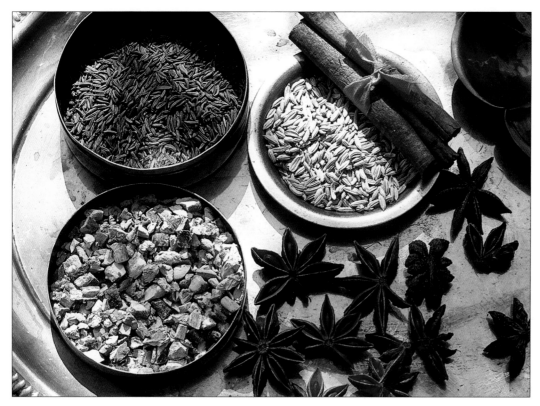

Spiced Lemon Verbena Mouthwash

Commercial antiseptic mouthwashes can upset the natural acid balance of the mouth. A herbal mouthwash is gentler and this one – made with lemon verbena – is particularly pleasant.

INGREDIENTS
5ml/1 tsp each ground nutmeg, ground cloves, cardamom pods and caraway seeds
small handful of fresh lemon verbena leaves or 15g/1/2 oz dried
600ml/1 pint/2¹/2 cups purified water
30ml/2 tbsp sweet sherry

Put the spices and lemon verbena into a pan with the water. Simmer for 30 minutes. Strain through a sieve lined with kitchen paper (kitchen towel), then add the sherry and pour into a clean bottle. To use, dilute 15–30ml/1–2 tbsp in a tumbler of water.

BELOW: Eat a sprig of parsley (LEFT) or watercress after a garlicky meal.

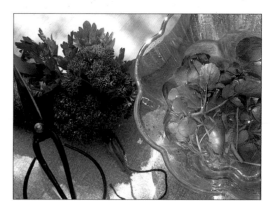

Sage and Myrrh Lotion for Mouth Ulcers

INGREDIENTS
15ml/1 tbsp dried sage
300ml/1/2 pint/11/4 cups boiling water
10ml/2 tsp tincture of myrrh

Pour the boiling water over the sage leaves in a jug (pitcher). Leave to stand for 20 minutes. Strain and mix in the tincture of myrrh. Use to rinse the mouth.

—SIMPLE TEETH CLEANSERS—
SAGE: Rub teeth with fresh sage leaves.
LEMON PEEL: Pare the peel off the fruit and rub over the teeth to remove stains.

ABOVE: Chewing seeds and spices to freshen the breath is a widespread custom in the East.

—SIMPLE BREATH FRESHENERS—
PARSLEY, WATERCRESS, MINT:
Chew the fresh leaves after eating a garlicky meal.
SEEDS OF FENNEL, STAR ANISE, ANGELICA, CARAWAY, CALAMUS ROOT, CINNAMON STICK, OR CLOVES: Suck or chew after a meal.
ROSEWATER: Dilute half-and-half with water for rinsing the mouth.
LAVENDER INFUSION: Make with 15ml/ 1 tbsp dried lavender in 300ml/ 1/2 pint/11/4 cups water and use as an oral rinse.

POT-POURRI

Natural plant fragrances induce a sense of well-being. They are a much healthier way to scent a room, or mask odours, than chemical air fresheners, some of which have recently been implicated in otherwise unexplained headaches and general debilitation in susceptible people.

Although commercially made pot-pourris are widely available, they are often artificially coloured and have a harsh, synthetic perfume which does little to restore and refresh the spirit. Making your own pot-pourri is fun, creative and couldn't be easier, using wholesome, naturally scented plants and essential oils.

Roses, pinks, bergamot (flowers and leaves), chamomile, peonies, jasmine, borage and lavender are among the most suitable flowers. For herbs, choose from lemon verbena, lemon balm, mint, basil, marjoram, thyme, rosemary and angelica seeds and leaves. If you do not grow these plants in your garden, you can buy the dried ingredients from specialist suppliers.

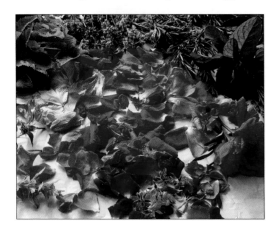

Gathering the Flowers and Herbs

When picking plants from the garden for pot-pourri, always choose a dry day. Roses, especially, tend to discolour and go mouldy if gathered when they are wet.

Drying

To dry roses, pull the petals apart and spread them on newspaper in an airing-cupboard, or in a dry warm room. Do not dry in direct sunlight, which will bleach the petals. Green herbs can be dried in the same way or tied in bunches and hung up in a warm, dry and airy place.

Spices, Oils and Fixatives

Spices ensure a lasting fragrance in the pot-pourri. Choose from allspice, cinnamon, nutmeg, cloves and ground coriander.

Plant essential oils complement and enhance the scent of the dried plants. Use high quality essential oils, rather than a cheap fragrance oil.

Ground orris root, made from the rhizome of the Florentine iris, is the best fixative, helping to preserve the overall scent of the mixture.

There are lots of recipes for pot-pourri, or you can experiment and make up your own.

LEFT: Rose petals have always been a top choice for pot-pourri. Mix them with plenty of dried green herbs for a natural, aromatic fragrance.

RIGHT: Spices, essential oil and ground orris root add to the scent of dried herbs and flowers.

Rose Pot-pourri
INGREDIENTS
3 cups dried rose petals
2 cups mixed dried flowers
15ml/1 tbsp dried lavender
1 cup mixed dried herbs: mint, marjoram, thyme and angelica
5ml/1 tsp cloves
2.5ml/¹⁄₂ tsp ground allspice
10ml/2 tsp ground orris root
5 drops bergamot essential oil
5 drops sandalwood essential oil

Combine all the ingredients, mix thoroughly and put them in an airtight container. Leave in a dry, warm place for 2–3 weeks. Shake the container occasionally during this time.

OPPOSITE: Pot-pourri soon loses its fragrance if constantly exposed to light and air. Keep it in a bowl with a lid, uncovering it when you want to scent the room.

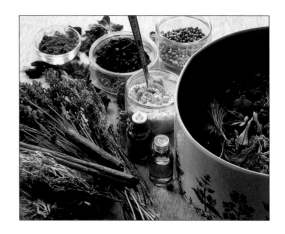

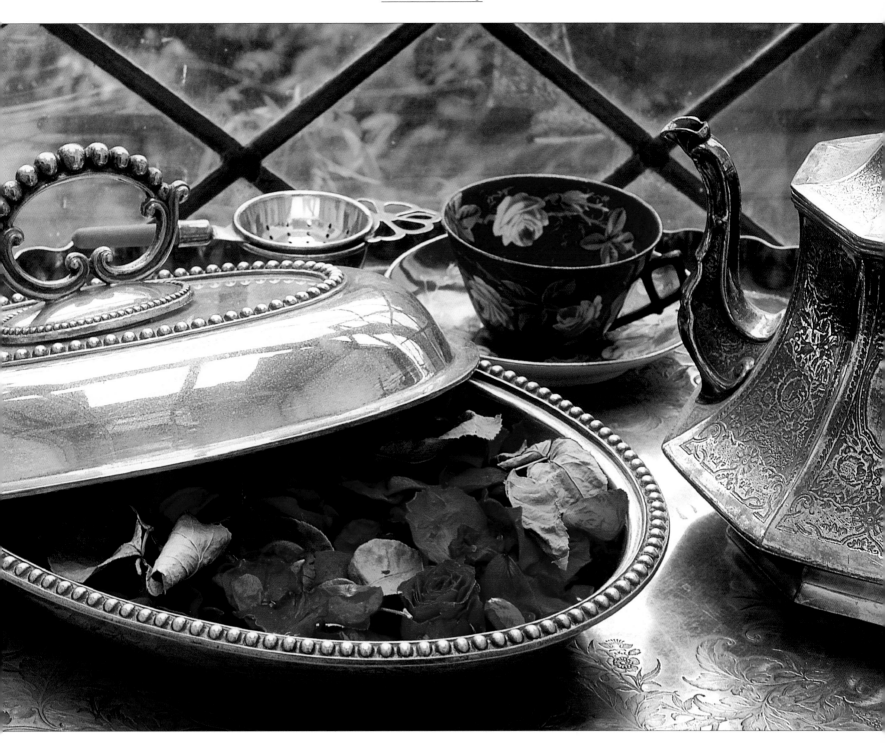

POMANDERS

Until well into the 17th century, no self-respecting apothecary would have been without his favourite formula for a pomander. This was due to a widely held belief in the power of fragrance to combat disease. The original pomanders were composed of strong-smelling substances usually of animal origin, chiefly civet, musk and ambergris, along with pulverized herbs and essences in a base of aromatic resin, with a "secret" ingredient, such as ground pearls, thrown in for good measure.

These exotic concoctions, often encased in jewelled holders, were much sought after as protection against the plague and other deadly infections. They were also extremely expensive. The cheaper alternative was an apple or, more effectively, an orange stuffed with a mixture of spices. This has stood the test of time as the ever-popular "clove-orange" pomander.

Citrus pomanders are well worth making for their relaxing fragrance or to keep in a cupboard to deter moths and insects. Well-made pomanders will keep their scent for many years.

Oranges are traditionally used as a base, but you can also use other citrus fruits such as lemons or you can make miniature pomanders from kumquats.

YOU WILL NEED
6–8 kumquats
knitting needle
25g/1oz cloves
10ml/2 tsp ground cinnamon
5ml/1 tsp ground orris root

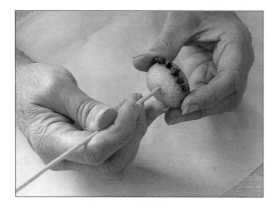

1 Using a knitting needle, pierce a row of holes in the skin of the fruit for the cloves.

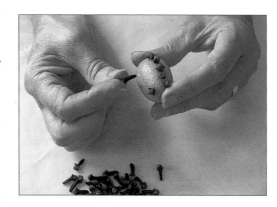

2 Press a clove into each hole, either covering the fruit completely or leaving gaps between the rows.

RIGHT: Kumquats make delightful miniature pomanders, instead of the traditional orange. They would also make a lovely gift.

OPPOSITE: Once dry, pomanders will have shrunk in size and should be totally hard.

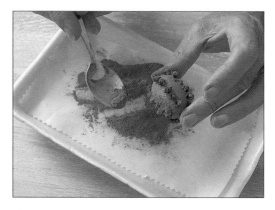

3 Mix the cinnamon and ground orris root together on a piece of greaseproof (waxed) paper. Roll the clove-studded kumquats in the mixture, tapping off any excess. Put them on a small cardboard tray and leave in a warm place, such as an airing-cupboard, until completely dried out. This will take 2–3 weeks (5–6 weeks for large oranges).

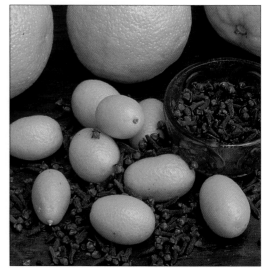

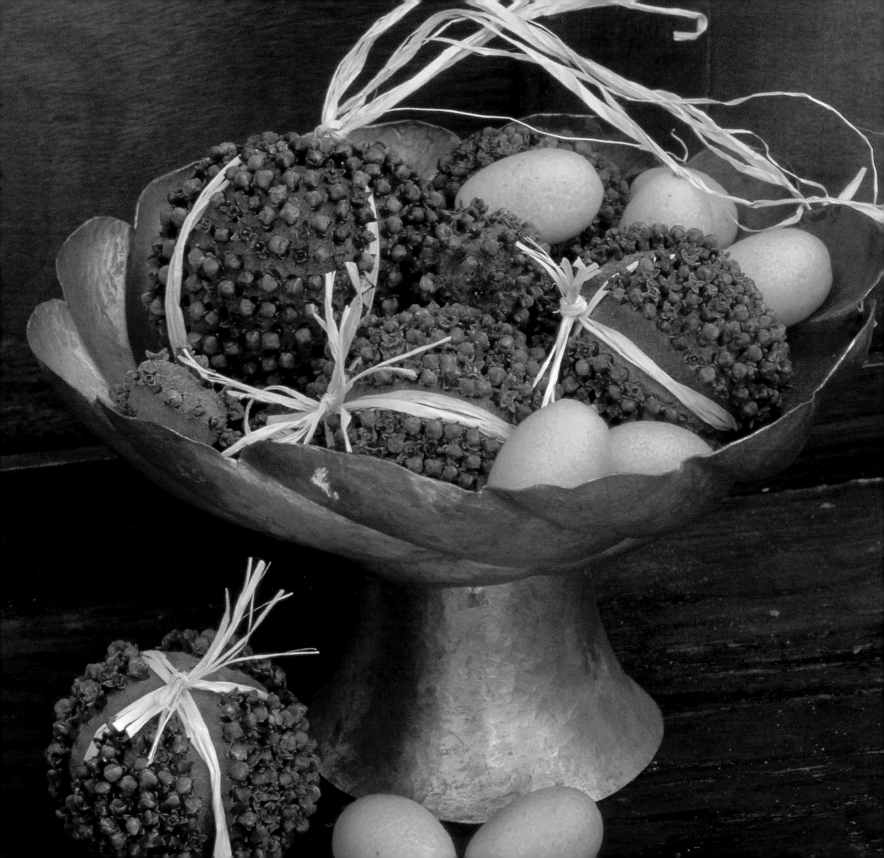

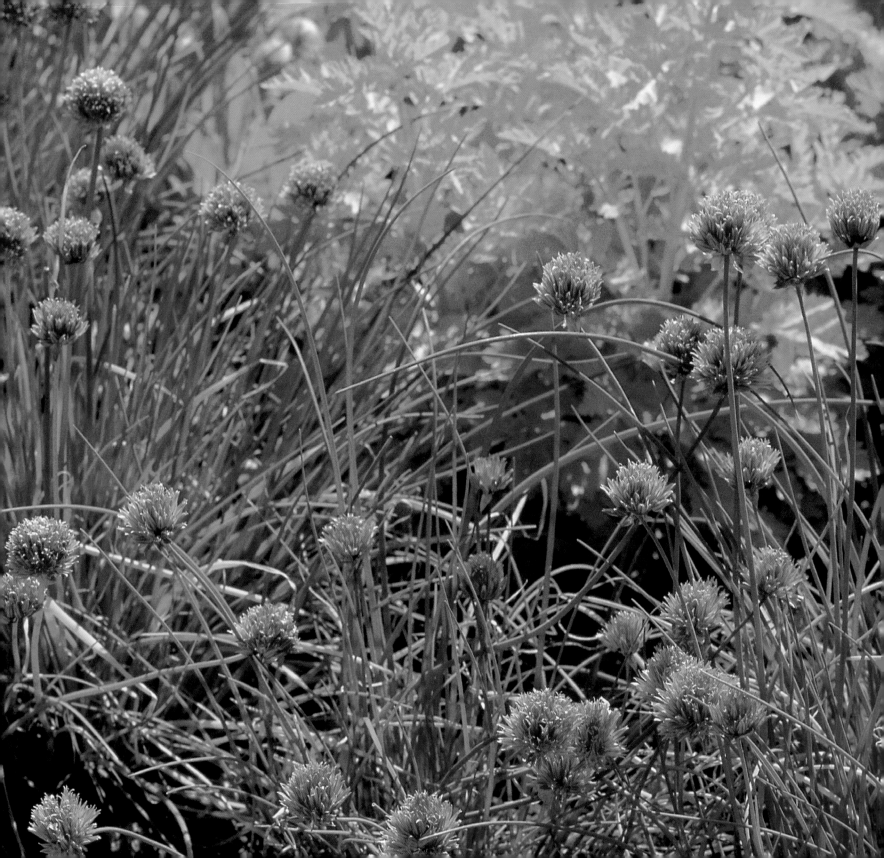

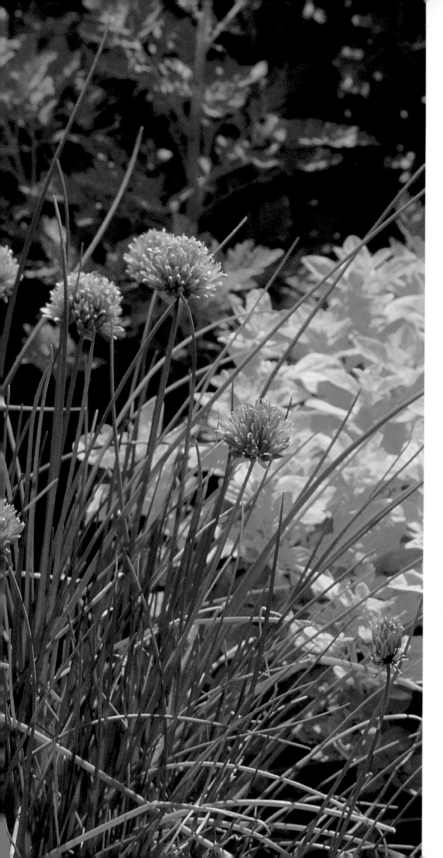

CHAPTER FIVE

GUIDE TO INGREDIENTS

―――――

*"O MICKLE IS THE POWERFUL GRACE THAT LIES
IN PLANTS, HERBS, STONES, AND THEIR TRUE QUALITIES."*
WILLIAM SHAKESPEARE, *ROMEO AND JULIET* (1599)

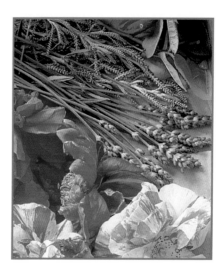

This chapter lists the herbs you will need for making remedies.
Most of the herbs are easy to grow. Spices, resins and other
ingredients used in the recipes are also briefly described and are
available from specialist suppliers.

*ABOVE: Garden plants, such as roses and lavender, form the basis of a
wide range of therapeutic preparations.*

*LEFT: Chives edge a herb garden that provides the ingredients for
home remedies.*

111

HERBS

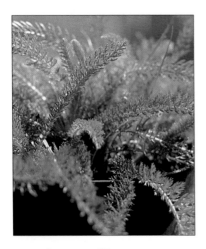

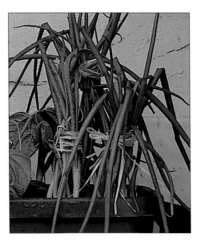

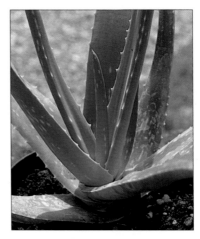

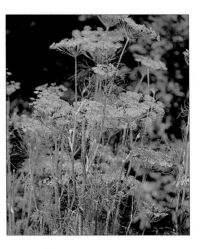

ACHILLEA MILLEFOLIUM
YARROW

The medicinal herb is the common weed, not an ornamental achillea. In folk medicine it was used to treat cuts and bleeding, harking back to its supposed origins as a wound-herb during the Trojan War – it is named for Achilles. It still has a place as a medicinal herb, but mainly in treating colds and catarrh.

PARTS USED: Leaves and flowering stems.

MEDICINAL: Take yarrow as an infusion for colds and allergic rhinitis, or put it into boiling water and inhale the steam. It can also be used for insect bites and headaches.

CAUTION: Yarrow can cause skin rashes and, if use is prolonged, increase the skin's sensitivity to sun. It should be avoided in pregnancy.

ALLIUM SATIVUM
GARLIC

Garlic was well known in the ancient world and was found in Tutankhamen's tomb. It has been widely valued as a medicinal and culinary herb over the centuries and has attracted many superstitions.

CULTIVATION: It needs rich, moist soil and plenty of sun. Propagate by planting individual cloves in autumn or winter.

PARTS USED: Bulbs.

MEDICINAL: Garlic has antibiotic properties and is used for bacterial infections, coughs and colds. It also helps stimulate the immune system and protect from infection, and lowers blood cholesterol. Eat it raw or cooked, or made into a syrup or tincture.

CULINARY: It adds flavour to a wide range of dishes and is an essential ingredient in many cuisines.

ALOE VERA SYN. ALOE
BARBADENSIS
ALOE VERA

A constituent of many modern cosmetic and pharmaceutical preparations, there is evidence that aloe vera was valued by the ancient Egyptians as a medicinal plant.

CULTIVATION: It does not withstand frost and in temperate climates can only be grown outdoors during the summer months. However, it makes a good houseplant.

PARTS USED: Sap and leaves.

MEDICINAL: The sap is anti-inflammatory and promotes healing. Slit the leaves and apply the gel directly to dry skin, eczema, irritations, rashes, burns, sunburn, insect bites and fungal infections such as athlete's foot.

ANETHUM GRAVEOLENS
DILL

Dill has been used as a medicine since earliest times. Pliny listed it as a prescription for many diseases, it appears in Anglo-Saxon herbals and was recommended by Culpeper (1650) "to stay hiccoughs … to expel wind, and the pains proceeding therefrom". In medieval times it was an anti-witchcraft herb.

CULTIVATION: An annual, dill is grown from seed, preferably sown *in situ* as it does not take kindly to transplantation and bolts.

PARTS USED: Leaves and seeds.

MEDICINAL: An ingredient of gripe water for colicky babies, the seeds are taken as a soothing, digestive tea. It has mildly sedative properties.

CULINARY: The leaves and seeds are widely used in cookery, especially in Scandinavian dishes, for flavouring seafood, eggs, salads and vegetables.

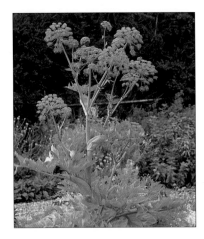

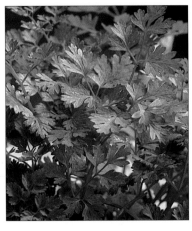

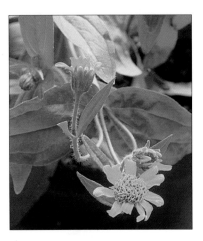

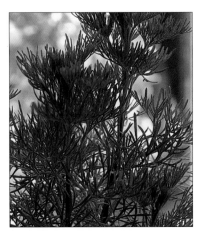

ANGELICA ARCHANGELICA
ANGELICA

The name reflects the esteem in which this plant was once held, both for its supposed powers against witchcraft and for its medicinal properties. Today its culinary uses are as important as the medicinal ones.

CULTIVATION: A statuesque biennial, which grows 1.5–2.4m/5–8ft tall, it does best in rich, moist soil. It is hardy and self-seeds freely.

PARTS USED: Leaves, stems, roots and seeds.

MEDICINAL: It has anti-inflammatory properties and is applied as a poultice for rheumatic pains and to ease sunburn. An infusion of the seeds or leaves makes a tea for indigestion. Chinese angelica *(A. sinensis)* has tonic properties and contains vitamins A and B.

CULINARY: Known primarily in candied form, the young fresh stems reduce acidity when cooked with rhubarb and other sour fruits.

AROMATIC: Dried for pot-pourri, the leaves retain a good colour.

ANTHRISCUS CEREFOLIUM
CHERVIL

Introduced to Britain by the Romans, this herb is now naturalized in many parts of the world. It is primarily a culinary herb, much used in France, with a subtle, anise flavour.

CULTIVATION: An annual, it is easy to grow from seed. Successional sowing ensures a supply over most months of the year. It does not transplant well, so grow it in containers, or sow straight into the ground.

PARTS USED: Leaves.

MEDICINAL: It has tonic, blood-cleansing properties and is also a digestive.

CULINARY: Add it to egg and fish dishes, salads and sauces. An essential ingredient of *fines herbes*.

ARNICA MONTANA
ARNICA (LEOPARD'S BANE)

Of north European origin, arnica was a popular medicinal plant in sixteenth-century Germany and is still widely used there to alleviate heart conditions.

CULTIVATION: Being an alpine, it prefers cool, well-drained soil. It is propagated by seed or division.

PARTS USED: Flowers and roots.

MEDICINAL: It is mainly used as an ointment for bruises and sprains and is also made into a homeopathic remedy.

CAUTION: Arnica can be poisonous if taken internally. Repeated external use may cause an allergic reaction. Never use it on broken skin.

ARTEMISIA ABROTANUM
SOUTHERNWOOD

The whole plant has a delightful, fresh lemony scent. It has insect-repellent properties and was known in France as *garde robe*, a reference to its use in sachets to keep moths out of the wardrobe. It was also frequently included in posies carried to ward off infection.

CULTIVATION: A shrubby perennial, which grows to 1m/3ft, southernwood makes an ideal hedge in the herb garden. It will grow in any soil, but prefers a sunny position. It is easy to propagate from cuttings.

PARTS USED: Leaves.

MEDICINAL: It has antiseptic properties and is used in preparations for dandruff and hair loss.

AROMATIC: Leaves are dried to go in insect-repellent pot-pourris.

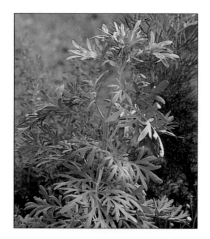

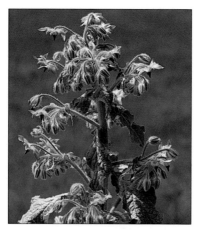

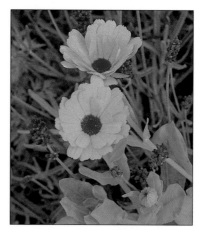

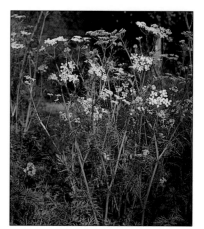

ARTEMISIA ABSINTHUM
WORMWOOD

In ancient Greece and Rome worm-wood was thought to be an effective antidote to poison by hemlock. Its power as an insect repellent was well recognized. Thomas Tusser, in his rhyming calender of garden tasks (1577), recommended it for getting rid of fleas, adding the couplet,

"What saver is better, if physick
be true,
For places infected than Wormwood
and Rue".

CULTIVATION: A silvery-leaved shrub which reaches 1m/3ft, it grows in any well-drained soil and is easily propagated by division.
PARTS USED: Leaves.
MEDICINAL: It has antiseptic and antibacterial properties. As an infusion it makes an insect-repellent lotion.
CAUTION: It should not be used in any form during pregnancy.

BORAGO OFFICINALIS
BORAGE

Borage, with its blue star-shaped flowers, has long been linked with courage and cheerfulness, and modern research indicates that it stimulates the adrenal glands, encouraging the flow of adrenaline. It contains vitamin C, calcium and potassium.
CULTIVATION: An annual, it is easy to grow from seed in any well-drained soil, but the plants will be bigger in moist soil. It often self-seeds.
PARTS USED: Leaves, flowers, seeds, essential oil.
MEDICINAL: Borage is a traditional ingredient of cough syrups. Make the leaves and flowers into a tea for anxiety and depression, or an infusion for soothing irritated skin.
CULINARY: Add flowers to salads and teas, leaves and flowers to wine and other drinks.

CALENDULA OFFICINALIS
MARIGOLD (POT MARIGOLD)

The bright orange heads of marigolds are a cheering sight in any herb garden and their habit of opening only to the sun, dutifully closing as shadows lengthen, was noted by the early herbalists. In earlier times they were dried for adding to winter broths, but they have little flavour and their culinary uses are perhaps less important today than the healing properties of the petals.
CULTIVATION: Easy to raise from seed, marigolds flower more prolifically in relatively poor soil.
PARTS USED: Flowers and essential oil.
MEDICINAL: The flowers have anti-inflammatory, antiseptic and healing properties, useful for skin irritations and wounds. The essential oil is antifungal, but not widely produced: a vegetable oil infused with the petals can be used instead of adding calendula oil to remedies.
CULINARY: Add petals to salads.
CAUTION: Do not confuse pot marigolds with French marigolds, *Tagetes* spp., which are toxic.

CARUM CARVI
CARAWAY

Caraway seed has been an ingredient of food and medicine since earliest times and was popular in ancient Rome and Greece.
CULTIVATION: A biennial, caraway is easy to grow from seed sown in spring or autumn. It flowers in its second year, when the seed-heads can be collected and hung to dry. It prefers full sun and well-drained soil.
PARTS USED: Leaves and seeds.
MEDICINAL: The seed on its own, or mixed with fennel, makes a digestive tea. Seeds can be chewed after meals to freshen the breath.
CULINARY: The young leaves have a milder taste than the seeds and can be added to salads or vegetable dishes. Use the seeds in cakes, breads, soups, stir-fry dishes, baked and stewed fruit.

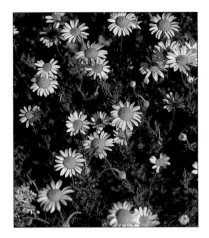

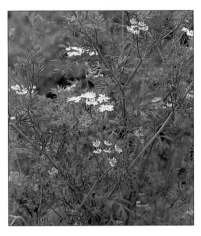

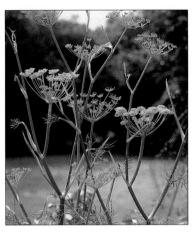

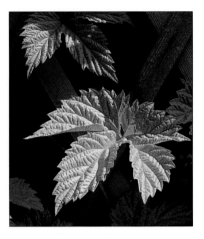

CHAMAEMELUM NOBILE
CHAMOMILE

Chamomile has an ancient pedigree, being one of the herbs in the Anglo-Saxon Nine Herbs Charm. The whole plant has a fresh, apple scent, especially after rain.

CULTIVATION: *C. nobile* is a perennial. It needs light, well-drained, but reasonably moist soil. Propagate by division in spring.

PARTS USED: Flowers.

MEDICINAL: Taken as a tea for digestive upsets and insomnia, soothing chamomile also has many uses in beauty treatments.

CORIANDRUM SATIVUM
CORIANDER

Grown in ancient Egypt and China over 5,000 years ago, coriander has remained a top culinary herb ever since. It is also an important aromatic, prized in perfumery, and a minor medicinal herb.

CULTIVATION: A hardy annual, it is grown from seed sown in early spring. It does not transplant well and often bolts quickly if the weather is hot and dry at the seedling stage.

PARTS USED: Leaves, seeds and essential oil.

MEDICINAL: It has digestive properties. The seeds can be chewed as a breath freshener. The essential oil is antifungal and antibacterial.

CULINARY: The leaves and seeds are widely used in Middle Eastern and Indian cookery, and the seeds in desserts, cakes and bread.

AROMATIC: The seeds are added to pot-pourri.

FOENICULUM VULGARE
FENNEL

Fennel's longstanding reputation for improving sight has its roots in the works of Pliny. William Coles in *The Art of Simpling* (1650) made the interesting connection of fennel with slimming. Recent research has found that part of the molecular structure of fennel resembles that of chemical amphetamines.

CULTIVATION: A tall perennial, reaching 1.5–1.8m/5–6ft, fennel is easy to grow and thrives in well-drained soil and full sun. It is propagated from seed.

PARTS USED: Leaves, seeds, stems, root and essential oil.

MEDICINAL: The seeds are made into a tea for flatulence and can be taken as an aid to losing weight. They are also chewed to freshen breath and made into a decoction to apply as a soothing compress for eyes.

CULINARY: Leaves and seeds have a sweetish, anise taste which complements fish and vegetable dishes.

HUMULUS LUPULUS
HOPS

The Romans ate young hop shoots as a vegetable but, although sometimes recommended as a medicinal herb, it was not widely grown in Britain until the sixteenth century, when it was first used in brewing beer. North American Indians recognized its sedative properties and also used it as a painkiller.

CULTIVATION: Male and female flowers are borne on separate plants of this hardy perennial climber. It requires rich, moist soil, and grows prolifically. Propagate from shoots in the spring. *H. l.* 'Aureus' is an ornamental golden-leaved cultivar.

PARTS USED: Female flowers.

MEDICINAL: The dried flowers have an antispasmodic action, which helps relieve muscle tension. Hops are put into pillows to aid restful sleep.

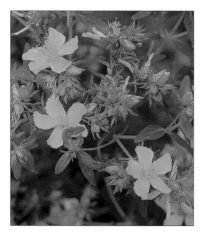

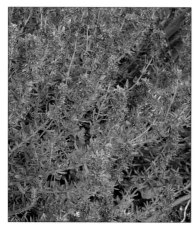

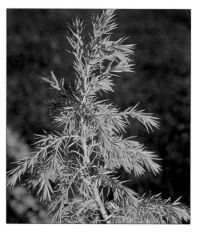

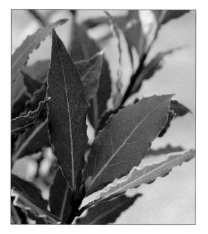

HYPERICUM PERFORATUM
ST JOHN'S WORT

Wild cousin of the garden hypericum, this plant has long enjoyed a
reputation as a herb with magical
properties. It is in fact a worthwhile
medicinal herb and is widely prescribed in Germany for depressive
disorders and heart conditions. It
has recently been the subject of an
extensive British study which found
that hypericum was as effective as
conventional drugs in treating
depression but, unlike them, completely devoid of side-effects.
CULTIVATION: A wild plant, it grows
in any soil and may be propagated
by division.
PARTS USED: Leaves and flowering
stems.
MEDICINAL: It has antibiotic and
antiviral properties, as well as being
an antidepressant. An infused oil is
made by steeping the flowers in a
vegetable carrier oil. Tea made from
the flowering stems is helpful for
nervous anxiety and tension
headaches.

HYSSOPUS OFFICINALIS
HYSSOP

There is some disagreement about
whether this is the biblical plant,
though the supplication "Purge me
with hyssop and I shall be clean"
does seem appropriate as it is fresh-
smelling and strongly aromatic. It
was a popular strewing herb.
CULTIVATION: A shrubby perennial,
hyssop has blue flower spires borne
in late summer. It grows well on
poor, dry soil, and should be pruned
hard in spring. It is easy to grow
from seed, but propagate pink-flow-
ered forms from cuttings.
PARTS USED: Leaves, flowering stems
and essential oil.
MEDICINAL: An anti-inflammatory,
expectorant herb, it can be taken
internally as an infusion for colds
and respiratory infections.
CULINARY: Use the leaves with dis-
cretion in casseroles and stews. Add
the flowers to salads.
AROMATIC: Hyssop has insect-repellent properties and can be used
dried in pot-pourri and sachets.

JUNIPERUS COMMUNIS
JUNIPER

The ancient Egyptians used juniper
for fumigation and in ritual cleansing ceremonies. Common juniper is
the medicinal plant: some cultivars
do not bear the all-important
berries.
CULTIVATION: A hardy shrub or small
tree, juniper grows in most soils.
PARTS USED: Fruits (berries) and
essential oil.
MEDICINAL: Taken internally, the
berries are beneficial for rheumatism, arthritis and gout. They can
also be applied externally, in the
form of massage oils, for rheumatism.
CULINARY: Juniper berries go well
with cabbage, pork and game. Use
in pickles, pork and soups.
CAUTION: *J. virginiana*, native to
America, and the red cedar oil it
produces, is extremely toxic if taken
internally.

LAURUS NOBILIS
BAY (BAY LAUREL, SWEET BAY)

One of the principle culinary herbs,
bay does have some medicinal uses
as well, and is prized for its year-
round availability. The leaves dry
well, with a strong, lasting flavour.
CULTIVATION: Although technically
frost hardy, bay should be given protection in hard winters. It makes an
attractive feature in a pot. It can be
propagated from cuttings, but they
are slow to establish.
PARTS USED: Leaves.
MEDICINAL: A digestive and appetite
stimulant. Bay can be applied externally as a compress for bruises and
sprains, or as a rinse for dandruff.
CULINARY: A prime ingredient of a
bouquet garni, bay adds flavour to
many dishes.
AROMATIC: Bay leaves are included in
tussie-mussies and pot-pourri.

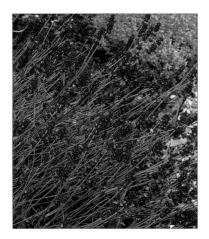

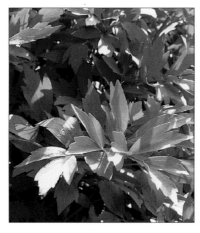

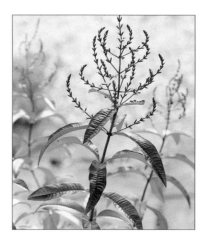

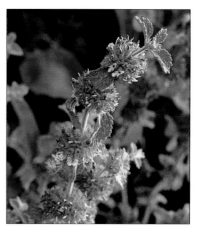

LAVANDULA SPP
LAVENDER

There are many species of lavender and many hybrids. For medicinal use *L. angustifolia* is best, though it is quite acceptable to use any of its varieties, such as 'Hidcote', 'Munstead', 'Nana alba' or 'Royal Purple'. *L. stoechas* was once widely used for medicinal purposes. The essential oil has many uses and is more important for medicinal and cosmetic recipes than the flowers.

CULTIVATION: A light, well-drained soil and full sun is best for lavenders. They should always be propagated from cuttings, as they do not come true from seed.

PARTS USED: Flowers and essential oil.

MEDICINAL: Lavender has antibacterial and antiseptic properties; it is a relaxant and a tonic for the nervous system. It can relieve headaches, soothe burns, bites and skin irritations and repel insects.

CULINARY: The flowers can be added to vinegar, and if used sparingly will add a distinctive flavour to jams, marmalade, biscuits and desserts.

LEVISTICUM OFFICINALE
LOVAGE

At one time lovage was widely used as a medicinal herb and more recently, in the nineteenth century, there was a popular cordial called "lovage", though it may well have included other herbs as well. It is now primarily a culinary herb.

CULTIVATION: It grows in any soil and is inclined to spread, making a wide clump and reaching 2m/6ft.

PARTS USED: Leaves.

MEDICINAL: Taken as a digestive for colic and flatulence, it also stimulates the appetite, increases perspiration and acts as a diuretic and expectorant.

CULINARY: Slightly salty, with a flavour like celery, it is an underused culinary herb. Use it in soups, stews and casseroles.

LIPPIA CITRIODORA SYN. *ALOYSIA TRIPHYLLA*
LEMON VERBENA

A native of South America, this aromatic plant keeps its fragrance for many years when dried.

CULTIVATION: Not fully hardy, it needs protection in severe winters. In warm climates it grows into a small tree up to 3m/10ft high. Despite its potential size, it grows well in containers. Cut it back hard in spring to encourage new shoots.

PARTS USED: Leaves and essential oil.

MEDICINAL: The essential oil is uplifting and antidepressant when inhaled. It is also antibacterial and insecticidal, but should never be applied directly to the skin as it may sensitize it to sunlight. The fresh leaves make a restorative tea.

AROMATIC: Add the dried leaves to pot-pourri.

MARRUBIUM VULGARE
HOREHOUND

This is the silvery-leaved white horehound, as opposed to *Ballota nigra,* the unpleasant smelling black horehound which does not have the same properties. This ancient herb was valued by the Egyptians and appears as an ingredient in a Roman recipe for an antidote to poison. Gerard recommended it for the same purpose, as well as for coughs and colds.

CULTIVATION: A hardy perennial, it grows in poor, dry soil. It can be propagated from seed, but is slow to germinate.

PARTS USED: Leaves and flowering stems.

MEDICINAL: It is used to make cough remedies.

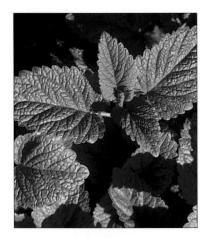

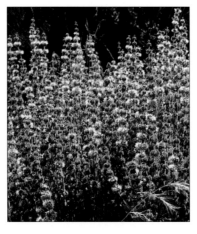

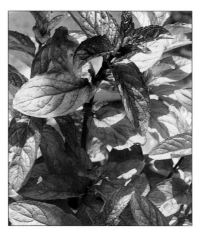

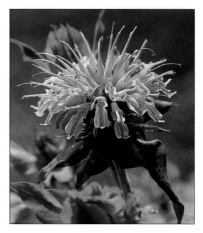

MELISSA OFFICINALIS
LEMON BALM

Often despised because it grows like a weed, lemon balm has a lovely, citrus scent, produces the essential oil melissa and has many medicinal, culinary and aromatic uses. The leaves do not keep the scent when dried and should be used fresh.

CULTIVATION: A hardy, herbaceous perennial, it grows in any soil, self-seeding freely.

PARTS USED: Leaves and esssential oil.

MEDICINAL: It has antidepressant properties and is relaxing and restorative to the nervous system, either taken as an infusion of the fresh leaves or inhaled as an essential oil. It can be used to relieve swellings and bruises, in the form of a compress, and to repel insects or relieve their bites.

CULINARY: The fresh leaves add a lemon flavour to fish and chicken dishes, soups, sauces and salads, wine and fruit cups.

MENTHA PULEGIUM
PENNYROYAL

Now valued chiefly for its aromatic properties, pennyroyal once enjoyed a high reputation as a medicinal herb and is extensively featured in the earliest herbals.

CULTIVATION: A species of mint, pennyroyal is undemanding and easy to grow. Propagate from runners.

PARTS USED: Leaves.

MEDICINAL: It is applied to skin irritations.

CULINARY: A pungently aromatic herb, pennyroyal is too strong for most tastes, although it is an ingredient of black pudding.

AROMATIC: It has insect-repellent properties and is reputed to be off-putting to ants. It is dried to put into sachets.

MENTHA SPP.
MINT

Mints have a wonderful scent and there are many species to choose from. Grow spearmint or applemint for cookery, peppermint for making tea, and eau-de-Cologne mint to scent the bath.

CULTIVATION: Grow mint in containers if you are worried about it spreading, or if your soil is so dry that it will not flourish – it needs damp soil. It is easy to propagate from runners and root cuttings.

PARTS USED: Leaves and essential oil.

MEDICINAL: It is an aromatic stimulant, with antibacterial properties. Peppermint is an excellent digestive, and can be taken as a tea to relieve colds and chills.

CULINARY: It is delicious in salads, sauces, and snipped over vegetables, especially potatoes.

MONARDA DIDYMA
BERGAMOT

Originally from North America, this lovely plant with soft, scented leaves and colourful flowers was made into a tea by North American Indians. 'Croftway Pink' and 'Cambridge Scarlet' are two of the most attractive cultivars, for tea and aromatic uses.

CULTIVATION: It will grow successfully only in damp soil. Dry conditions increase its tendency to suffer from mildew. Propagate by division.

PARTS USED: Flowers and leaves.

MEDICINAL: Taken as a tea for feverish colds, it also makes a reviving drink first thing in the morning.

AROMATIC: Use it in pot-pourri.

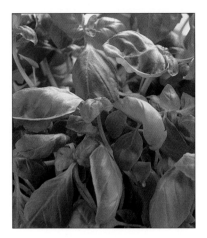 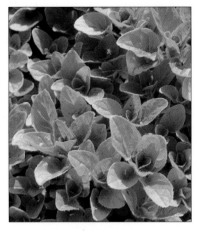 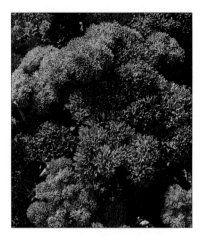 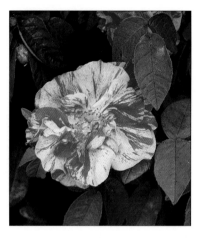

Ocimum Basilicum	***Origanum*** SPP.	***Petroselinum Crispum***	***Rosa*** SPP.
BASIL	MARJORAM	PARSLEY	ROSE

BASIL

Basil is a native of India, where it is a sacred plant. There are many species, including several attractive purple forms, but basil hybridizes easily, producing some odd variations. Rich in essential oils, it has a warm, aromatic scent.

CULTIVATION: As it is tender, it is grown as an annual in temperate regions. It prefers a moist but well-drained soil, and is best grown in a container.

PARTS USED: The whole herb and essential oil.

MEDICINAL: Basil has antiseptic properties and helps lift depression. Rub the fresh leaves on to insect bites; the essential oil, diluted in a carrier oil, makes an insect repellent. Use in steam inhalations for colds and catarrh.

CULINARY: It makes a delicious herb oil. Well-known for its affinity with tomatoes, basil is widely used in pasta dishes, salads and other Mediterranean cookery.

MARJORAM

Marjoram is chiefly used as a culinary herb, but it does have some medicinal applications and is also valued for its aromatic properties and essential oil. Pot marjoram *(O. onites)*, wild marjoram *(O. vulgaris)*, and sweet marjoram *(O. majorana)* are best for culinary and medicinal use.

CULTIVATION: Of the three species mentioned, *O. majorana* is half-hardy; the others tolerate frost. They need a well-drained soil, and are easy to propagate by division.

PARTS USED: Leaves, flowering stems, essential oil.

MEDICINAL: Take as a tea for headaches or use in a compress to relieve rheumatic pains and aching joints. The essential oil has a relaxing effect when inhaled.

CULINARY: Marjoram is good as a dried herb; it is much used in Greek and Italian cookery.

AROMATIC: Add to pot-pourri.

PARSLEY

The Greeks put parsley on their tombs and fed it to their chariot horses, but seldom ate it themselves. In seventeenth-century Europe, herbalists concluded it could be an antidote to poison and more recently it became a ubiquitous garnish, left on the side of everyone's plate. It does not have a directly medicinal action but its credentials as a highly nutritious culinary herb have now been firmly established. Both curly and flat-leafed parsley contain vitamins A and C, iron and antioxidants.

CULTIVATION: A biennial, parsley needs a well-worked, reasonably rich and moist soil if it is to flourish. It is grown from seed.

PARTS USED: Leaves and stalks.

CULINARY: Parsley complements many dishes and its mild and delicious flavour means it can be eaten in large quantities in dishes such as tabbouleh.

ROSE

Early herbals are full of rose recipes: medicinal, cosmetic, culinary and generally uplifting. Red rose petals were still listed in the British Pharmacopoeia as recently as the 1930s. The essential oil is highly complex, with over 300 chemical constituents. It has a gentle, therapeutic action on the skin, but is prohibitively expensive. *Rosa gallica officinalis* is known as the Apothecary's Rose, and was once widely used in medicinal preparations. Pictured above is *Rosa gallica versicolor*.

PARTS USED: Petals, hips and essential oil.

MEDICINAL: Rose acts as an anti-depressant when the essential oil is inhaled in steam or used in a massage oil. It also has an anti-inflammatory action in creams and lotions and is soothing to sensitive skin. The hips are made into cough syrups and are a valuable source of vitamin C.

CULINARY: Use the petals to flavour vinegar, conserves and desserts.

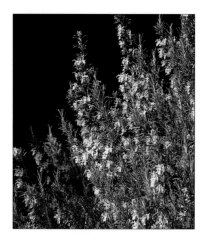

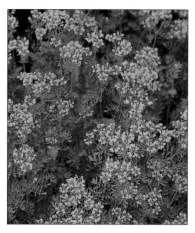

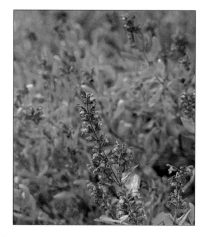

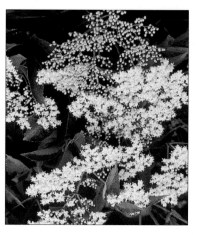

ROSMARINUS OFFICINALIS
ROSEMARY

Rosemary has a longstanding reputation for strengthening the memory. The essential oil was one of the first plant oils to be distilled in the fourteenth century and its bracing scent has a "head-clearing" quality. In modern herbal medicine it has an important place as an anti-depressant.

CULTIVATION: Although it stands up to frost when established, rosemary is not reliably hardy and needs protection in harsh winters. It grows best on light, free-draining soil and is propagated from cuttings.

PARTS USED: Leaves, flowering stems and essential oil.

MEDICINAL: It has restorative properties and can be taken as a tea for headaches, anxiety, tiredness and debilitation. Use the fresh leaves or the essential oil in steam inhalations for nervous exhaustion.

CULINARY: A traditional flavouring for lamb, it can also be added to herb oils and vinegars.

RUTA GRAVEOLENS
RUE

Early writers recommended rue as an antidote to poison. More sensibly, its insecticide properties were also recognized: dried rue was spread on the floor and rue-water sprinkled in houses to kill fleas.

CULTIVATION: It prefers light, well-drained soil. It can be propagated from seed or cuttings.

PARTS USED: Leaves and flowers.

AROMATIC: It is dried for inclusion in insect-repellent sachets.

CAUTION: Always wear gloves to handle rue as it can cause severe blistering.

SALVIA OFFICINALIS
SAGE

The Latin name is derived from *salvere,* "to save", a reference to its curative properties, and this common garden plant has many medicinal uses. Purple sage is sometimes said to be the more powerful for this purpose.

CULTIVATION: A native of the Mediterranean, sage grows best in light, free-draining soil. Purple sage is mostly hardy, but tricolour sage should be given winter protection against frost. Propagated from cuttings, or by layering.

PARTS USED: Leaves and essential oil.

MEDICINAL: Sage has antiseptic and antibacterial properties and is a traditional ingredient of cough, cold and respiratory remedies.

CULINARY: A popular culinary herb, it adds flavour to many dishes.

SAMBUCUS NIGRA
ELDER

Known as "the medicine chest of the country people", this common wayside tree, now largely ignored, was once revered. It attracted a wealth of superstitions and right across Europe was held to drive away evil spirits and guard against witchcraft.

PARTS USED: Flowers, berries and leaves.

MEDICINAL: The flowers are anti-catarrhal and, if taken as a tea or tincture before pollen counts rise, they may be helpful in reducing hayfever symptoms. They are also anti-inflammatory and soothing to sensitive or inflamed skin. The berries are rich in vitamins A and C, and both flowers and berries are made into cordials to take for colds. The leaves have insect-repellent properties.

CULINARY: The flowers have a delicious muscatel flavour and go well with gooseberries. Make them into fritters, ice-creams and sorbets.

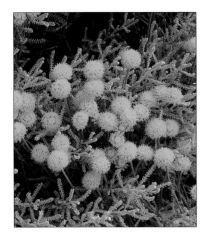

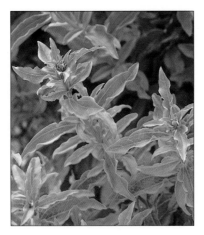

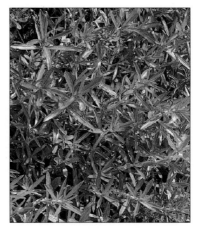

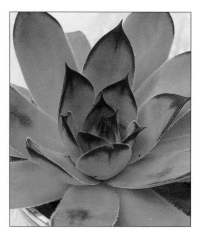

SANTOLINA CHAMAECYPARISSUS
COTTON LAVENDER

This silver-leafed herb (there are also some green varieties) grows wild on Mediterranean hillsides and came to Britain in the sixteenth century, featuring in the formal knot gardens popular at the time. It was also used as an insecticide and strewing herb.

CULTIVATION: A perennial, santolina prefers well-drained soil and full sun and needs little water. It does not survive well in harsh winters without protection. Trim frequently to keep it in shape.

PARTS USED: Leaves and flowering stems.

MEDICINAL: It has anti-inflammatory properties and can be used in poultices to treat minor skin irritations and insect bites.

AROMATIC: Strongly aromatic, with a clean "disinfectant" smell, it dries well for inclusion in pot-pourris and insect-repellent sachets.

SAPONARIA OFFICINALIS
SOAPWORT

Before the days of modern soap, this creeping plant, with its pretty pink flowers, was a valuable aid to cleanliness. The leaves and roots contain saponins, and when boiled or infused make a liquid which lathers when whisked or shaken. It has been found to be the best way of cleaning old tapestries and delicate fabrics which do not stand up to treatment with modern detergents.

CULTIVATION: A somewhat invasive wild plant with creeping roots, it flourishes in poor soil.

PARTS USED: Roots, stems, leaves and flowers.

COSMETIC: The fresh plant, including the root, is dug up to make a soapy liquid for washing the hair for those who prefer to avoid detergent-based shampoos.

SATUREJA HORTENSIS AND S. MONTANA
SAVORY, SUMMER AND WINTER

Enjoyed in Roman times for their flavour, both these herbs have a subtle, spicy scent and, as their name suggests, are ideal for culinary purposes. Savory was a "must-have" herb taken to America by British colonists.

CULTIVATION: Summer savory is an annual and winter savory a perennial that forms a low-growing clump. Both can be grown from seed and winter savory can also be increased by division.

PARTS USED: Leaves and essential oil.

MEDICINAL: The savories have antibacterial properties and an infusion can be used as an antiseptic gargle. They are also digestive and stimulating to the appetite.

CULINARY: The savories have an affinity with beans and flavour many egg, fish or meat dishes.

SEMPERVIVUM TECTORUM
HOUSELEEK

In medieval times this attractive succulent was grown on cottage roofs all over Europe, and the superstition arose that it gave protection from lightning strikes. It was also valued from earliest times as a medicinal plant for skin diseases. "Leek" in this context, comes from the Anglo-Saxon word for plant, *leac*.

CULTIVATION: It grows well in dry soil and spreads, but is not invasive. It is easy to propagate by separating the runners.

PARTS USED: Leaves.

MEDICINAL: Juice from the bruised or split leaves is applied to inflamed or irritated skin, burns, insect bites and stings.

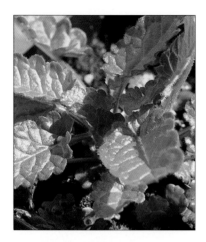

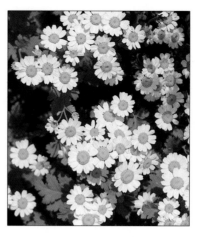

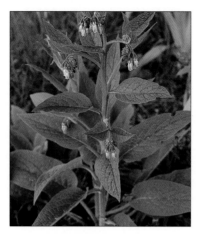

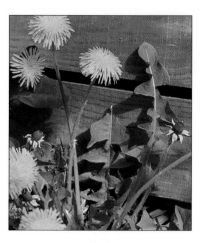

STACHYS OFFICINALIS
BETONY

Once a standard in all physic gardens, it was valued as a medicinal plant and was believed to have supernatural powers, with the ability to guard against evil spirits.

CULTIVATION: A wild plant, with a pretty fuschia-pink flower, it grows easily in ordinary dry soil.

PARTS USED: The whole plant.

MEDICINAL: It can be taken as a tea for tension headaches, but only in very small quantities. One or two leaves should be added to another herb tea, such as rosemary or St John's wort.

CAUTION: In large doses betony can cause vomiting and diarrhoea; avoid it in pregnancy.

SYMPHYTUM OFFICINALE
COMFREY

The old country name "knitbone" signals the healing properties of this useful herb. The rotted leaves make a good compost heap activator and organic garden fertilizer, rich in plant nutrients.

CULTIVATION: A tall perennial with a tough tap-root, comfrey needs plenty of room. It will grow anywhere and is hard to eradicate once established.

PARTS USED: Leaves and root.

MEDICINAL: The leaves contain a soothing, anti-inflammatory mucilage and are made into ointments and poultices to apply externally to wounds, abrasions and bruises.

CAUTION: Do not take comfrey internally.

TANACETUM PARTHENIUM SYN. *CHRYSANTHEMUM PARTHENIUM*
FEVERFEW

Feverfew came to prominence as a modern medicinal herb when it was found to be effective against migraine, but it was already being used for this purpose by herbalists in the sixteenth and seventeenth centuries.

CULTIVATION: A hardy perennial that self-seeds freely. Propagate from seed or by division in spring.

PARTS USED: Leaves.

MEDICINAL: It is taken internally for migraine and rheumatism, either as fresh leaves or a weak infusion with plenty of honey to disguise the bitter taste. Externally, as an infusion or tincture, it can be applied to insect bites.

CAUTION: Overuse can cause mouth ulcers or dermatitis if applied externally. Do not use it if you are pregnant.

TARAXACUM OFFICINALE
DANDELION

Dandelion leaves are strongly diuretic, hence their French name *pissenlit,* but their high vitamin and mineral content makes them a worthwhile tonic.

PARTS USED: Leaves and roots.

MEDICINAL: The leaves contain vitamins A, B, C and D, potassium, iron and other minerals, and are eaten young for their tonic properties – older, fully-grown leaves are too bitter. The roots have anti-rheumatic properties and are used commercially to make a pleasant-tasting coffee.

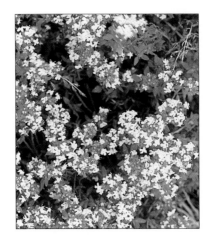

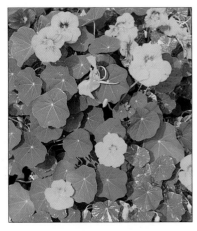

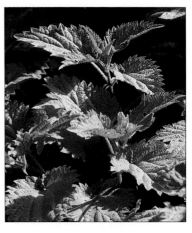

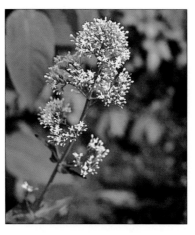

THYMUS VULGARIS AND *T. SERPYLLUM*
THYME

Recent research has linked thyme esssential oil with slowing the ageing process, and a commercial product, based on thyme oil, is now available which claims to help maintain eye and brain function. It is one of the most useful herbs in the garden, with many medicinal uses.

CULTIVATION: As a herb of Mediterranean hillsides, it prefers light, well-drained soil and does not flourish if its roots are waterlogged or in very harsh winters. Propagate from cuttings.

PARTS USED: Leaves and essential oil.

MEDICINAL: It is both antiseptic and antibacterial and is used in sore throat remedies, for coughs and colds, and to heal wounds.

CULINARY: A useful seasoning herb for low-fat, low-salt diets, it is a component of the classic *bouquet garni,* and is added as a flavouring to soups, stews, casseroles and other slow-cooked dishes.

TROPAEOLUM MAJUS
NASTURTIUM

This now familiar garden flower came to Europe in the sixteenth century from South America.

CULTIVATION: A half-hardy annual, it is easy to grow from seed and makes a colourful subject for a container. It likes moisture but plenty of sun, and flowers best in poor soil.

PARTS USED: Flowers, leaves, and seeds.

MEDICINAL: It has antiseptic properties and is used in hair preparations for dandruff and dry scalp. It has also been claimed to help reduce hair loss.

CULINARY: The leaves, which have a peppery flavour, contain vitamin C and both leaves and flowers can be added to salads. The seeds are pickled as a substitute for capers.

URTICA DIOICA
NETTLES

Stinging nettles have a venerable place in folk medicine. The nettle was one of the sacred herbs invoked in the ancient Nine Herbs Charm. The tenth-century *Leech Book of Bald* advises, "Take nettles and seethe them in oil, smear and rub all thy body therewith; the cold will depart away". Nettles still have a worthy place in herbal medicine.

PARTS USED: Leaves.

MEDICINAL: Rich in iron, they make an excellent tonic, and as they also contain plenty of vitamin C, the iron is properly absorbed by the body. It is also thought that nettles may help to relieve arthritis and gout by clearing uric acid from the system. They are included in hair rinses for treating dry scalp, dandruff and hair loss.

VALERIANA OFFICINALIS
VALERIAN

Valerian is named in Anglo-Saxon herbals of the eleventh century, when its tranquillizing properties were clearly appreciated. This is still its main use in herbal medicine today.

CULTIVATION: It grows in most conditions, though its preference is for a moist soil. Propagate it by division.

PARTS USED: Root, dried or fresh.

MEDICINAL: Use in an infusion or a decoction of the roots for anxiety, nervous tension and insomnia.

SPICES AND OTHER INGREDIENTS

—Spices—

CARAWAY SEEDS
CARUM CARVI

The seeds are digestive when taken as a tea or added to food.

CAYENNE PEPPER
CAPSICUM FRUTESCENS

The ground form of the hot, red cayenne chilli. A tonic for the nervous system, it also has antibacterial and antiseptic properties, stimulates the circulation, increases blood flow and encourages perspiration. It contains vitamins A, B and C. It is good for colds and sore throats, but excessive doses are harmful.

BELOW: Many spices have antiseptic and antibacterial properties.

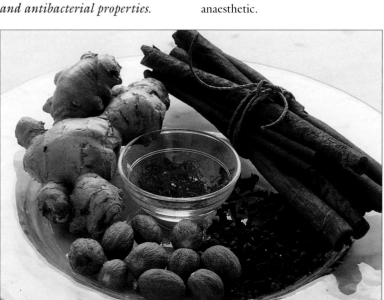

CINNAMON
CINNAMONUM SPP.

Cinnamon sticks are made from the rolled inner bark of a tropical tree. It is also used in ground form. Pungent and warming, cinnamon is good for colds and has digestive properties. The essential oil is antibacterial and antifungal.

CLOVES
SYZYGIUM AROMATICUM

Cloves are the dried immature flower buds of a small tropical tree. They are stimulating, warming, have digestive properties and help prevent nausea. The essential oil is applied externally to relieve toothache. They are also antiseptic, and slightly anaesthetic.

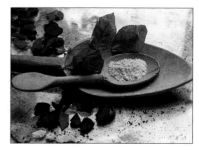

ABOVE: Orris root is the ground rhizome of the Florentine iris.

GINGER
ZINGIBER OFFICINALIS

Ginger is a plant of tropical forests. The rhizome is used fresh or dried and ground. It is often preserved in syrup or crystallized and is an essential ingredient of Eastern cookery. It stimulates circulation, prevents nausea and is used in cold remedies.

MACE AND NUTMEG
MYRISTICA FRAGRANS

Both spices are obtained from the same tree: mace is the outer casing of the fruit and nutmeg is the kernel. Nutmeg has digestive properties and helps prevent nausea and vomiting. The essential oil is added to a carrier oil as a massage for rheumatism. Do not take nutmeg internally in large quantities.

ORRIS ROOT

The ground rhizome of the Florentine iris, it is creamy-white and smells faintly of violets. It is a fixative for giving pot-pourri a lasting scent.

SLIPPERY ELM

The powdered bark of the elm tree *Ulmus fulva*, native to North America, it has strengthening and healing properties and is used in poultices. It can also be taken internally, mixed with water, for stomach upsets.

—Gums and Resins—

BENZOIN

An aromatic resin from the styrax tree, benzoin has preservative, antiseptic qualities. It is available as a tincture or in ground form for adding to creams and ointments.

FRANKINCENSE

This important component of incense is the gum resin of *Boswellia thurifera*, a tree native to Africa and the Middle East. The essential oil has warming, relaxing properties. It is also available in granular form for adding to pot-pourri.

MYRRH

Used by the ancient Egyptians in mummification, myrrh is the gum resin of a small shrub native to the Middle East, Somalia and Ethiopia. It is antifungal, antiseptic, helps clear catarrh and stimulates the immune system. Its preservative qualities make it useful in creams and lotions and for fixing the scent of pot-pourri. It is available as a tincture or in ground or granular form, or as an essential oil.

—Minerals—
Borax
A mineral deposited on the shores of alkaline lakes, borax has cleaning properties. It also acts as an emulsifier to bind oils and water together when making creams.

Fuller's Earth
A clay-like substance – hydrous aluminium silicate – it was formerly used to "full" or finish woollen cloth by cleaning it of oil and grease. Rich in minerals, it has excellent drawing and stimulating properties for poultices and face masks.

—Oils and Waxes—
Beeswax
Beeswax is naturally yellow: white beeswax is bleached and treated. It is

Below: Almond and other vegetable oils.

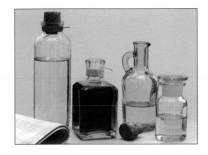

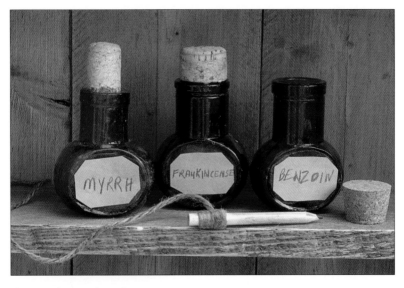

Above: Aromatic resins act as preservatives in lotions.

used as an emulsifier for oil and water mixtures and has a high melting point.

Cocoa Butter
This is the fat from the cocoa bean. Cream-coloured and smelling faintly of chocolate, it is rich, oily and moisturizing.

Coconut Oil
Extracted from the white flesh, it is rich and moisturizing to the skin. At room temperature and below it is solid but melts when lukewarm.

Emulsifying Wax
Also available in ointment form, this wax is made from ceto stearyl alcohol and lauryl sulphate. Lanolin makes an organic substitute. The ointment is easier to use and melts more readily.

Glycerine
Glycerine is a sticky, odourless and colourless liquid, which is soluble in water. It attracts and holds water and is very lubricating.

Lanolin
The sebum from sheeps' wool, lanolin has a thick, sticky consistency and can be used as an organic alternative to emulsifying wax. It does not have such a pleasant texture, however, and can cause allergies in susceptible people. Hydrous lanolin contains added water, anhydrous lanolin does not and is thicker in texture.

Petroleum Jelly
A mineral jelly with lubricating properties. It is not easily absorbed by the skin, but forms a protective layer over it and makes a good base for ointments.

Right: A few basic ingredients are needed for home remedies.

Vegetable Oils
Almond, olive, safflower and sunflower oils make suitable base oils. Wheatgerm oil, rich in minerals and vitamin E, is added in small quantities for its properties, rather than as a base or carrier oil.

—Essential Oils—
Essential oils, also known as "volatile oils" because they readily evaporate, are quite distinct from fatty, vegetable oils. They are not greasy, often colourless, and are contained in minute droplets in the roots, leaves, stems, flowers, bark or resins of plants. Their chemical structure is complex and gives the plant its characteristic odour. Most are extracted by steam distillation or by the use of volatile solvents.

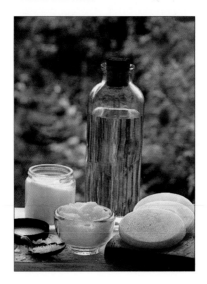

AILMENTS AND TREATMENTS

Ailments may not necessarily be cured by the treatments suggested here, but they may at least be alleviated. Serious or chronic conditions should always be referred to a medical practitioner.

—Aches and Pains—

ARTHRITIS AND RHEUMATISM: Angelica, marjoram as compress; juniper berries, garlic taken internally, or applied in massage oil; eucalyptus in bath oil.

ARTHRITIS AND GOUT: nettles in tea, soup or as a vegetable.

SPRAINS AND STRAINS: bay as compress; arnica, comfrey, *Aloe vera*, pot marigold, yarrow in ointment or poultice; valerian compress.

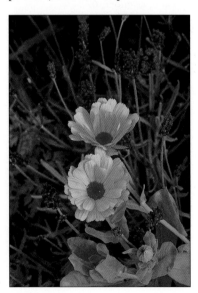

—Eye Complaints—

SORE, ITCHING EYES: fennel, chamomile, rose as compress.

—Headaches—

TENSION AND OTHER HEADACHES: St John's wort, marjoram, rosemary, yarrow as infusions; lavender as compress; lavender oil inhaled.

MIGRAINES: feverfew taken internally.

—Digestive Problems—

DIGESTIVE UPSETS: dill, angelica, caraway, chervil, coriander, fennel, lovage as tea, or added to food; chamomile as tea.

NAUSEA: cinnamon, cloves, ginger, nutmeg taken internally.

—Nervous Disorders—

ANXIETY AND DEPRESSION: borage, rosemary, St John's wort, valerian, basil, lemon verbena, lemon balm as tea; basil, bergamot, chamomile, frankincense, jasmine, lavender, neroli, rose, sandalwood, thyme, ylang-ylang as essential oils to inhale.

INSOMNIA: chamomile, dill, elderflower, lavender, limeflower, valerian as tea; hops in pillow; violet tincture taken internally; lavender, juniper, chamomile, marjoram, neroli, rose, sandalwood as essential oils to inhale.

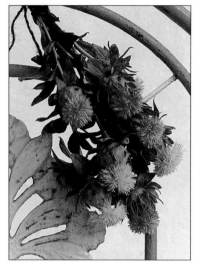

—Respiratory Problems—

COUGHS: borage, hyssop, thyme, horehound, sage as gargles or teas; linctus, garlic, ginger as decoctions.

COLDS: elderflower, horehound, sage, peppermint, thyme as tea; elderberries as cordial; garlic, ginger as decoction or syrup; cayenne, cinnamon taken internally; camphor, eucalyptus, lavender inhaled.

RHINITIS: elderflower tea, tincture or cordial; sage tea.

SINUSITIS: eucalyptus, basil, hyssop, juniper, sage, thyme, cayenne, cinnamon, eucalyptus, inhaled.

SORE THROAT: cayenne, hyssop, sage, savory, thyme as a tea or as a gargle.

—Skin and Hair Complaints—

BURNS: *Aloe vera*, houseleek, fresh leaf or lotion externally; pot marigold cream; lavender essential oil externally.

BITES AND STINGS: *Aloe vera*, houseleek, lemon balm, basil, onion externally; pot marigold, comfrey, yarrow as ointment; lavender oil, witch hazel.

BRUISES: comfrey, arnica, yarrow as poultice or ointment.

CUTS AND ABRASIONS: pot marigold, comfrey, thyme, sage as compress or ointment; tea tree oil externally.

FUNGAL INFECTIONS: tea tree oil, *Aloe vera*, myrrh externally.

SPOTS: garlic, tea tree oil, externally.

SUNBURN: angelica, *Aloe vera* as poultice; pot marigold, witch hazel.

RASHES AND SKIN IRRITATIONS: *Aloe vera*, houseleek as poultices; pot marigold as cream.

DANDRUFF, DRY SCALP: bay, nettles, rosemary, southernwood as rinses.

HAIR LOSS: nasturtium, nettle as rinses.

INDEX

aches and pains, 89, 126
ailments, 126
aloe vera, 35, 66, 112
angelica, 74, 105, 106, 113
antioxidants, 42-3
anxiety, herb teas, 51
applemint, 18
arnica, 66, 113

basil, 22, 44, 45, 66, 119
bath bags, 88-9
bath oils and lotions, 90-1
bay, 11, 46, 83, 116
beeswax, 67, 96, 125
benzoin, 124
bergamot, 32, 51, 118
betony, 122
bites, 34-5
blackberry vinegar, 47
borage, 32, 42, 56, 60, 114
borax, 125
bottles, sterilizing, 52
breath fresheners, 105
bruises, 34-5, 70-1, 74

candles, insect-repellent, 85
caraway, 32, 105, 114, 124
carrot poultices, 74
cayenne pepper, 42, 45, 124
chamomile, 17, 32, 36, 50, 51, 76,
  80, 89, 92, 98, 99, 115
chervil, 113
chives, 14, 23, 111
cider vinegar, 46
cinnamon, 46, 105, 106, 124
cloves, 108, 124
cocoa butter, 125
coconut oil, 91, 125

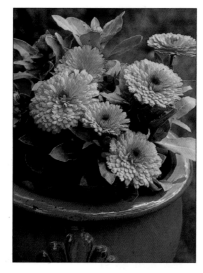

colds, 28-9, 50, 58, 60, 72
comfrey, 34, 70, 74, 89, 93, 122
composts, containers, 18
compresses, 76
containers, 18-19
cordials, 59
coriander, 59, 115
cotton lavender, 33, 83,121
coughs, 50, 60
cuttings, 15-16

dandelion, 42, 56, 122
dandruff, 99
depression, herb teas for, 51
design, herb gardens, 11
diet, 42-3
digestive problems, 50, 126
dill, 32, 50, 112
dividing plants, 14
dock leaves, 66
drying herbs, 20-1, 106

early morning teas, 51
eau-de-Cologne mint, 18
elderberries, 42, 59, 120
elderflowers, 50, 51, 59, 63, 94,
  96-7, 120
emulsifying wax, 125
essential oils, 66, 125
  bath oils, 90-1
  burners, 78-9
  steam inhalants, 77
eucalyptus, 72
eye complaints, 76, 126

face treatments, 92-3
fennel, 50, 76, 105, 115
fertilizers, containers, 19
feverfew, 30, 122
first aid, 66
foot baths, 102-3
Four Thieves Vinegar, 46
fragrant basket for relaxation, 26-7
frankincense, 80, 124
Fuller's earth, 125

gargles, 61
garlic, 42, 45, 54, 58, 66, 72, 112
ginger, 42, 60, 124
glycerine, 125
growing herbs, 9-39

hair care, 36-7, 99, 126
hand treatments, 100-1
hanging baskets, 26-7
harvesting herbs, 20
headaches, 30-1, 51, 76, 126
herbals, 6
hops, 80, 115
horehound, 28, 34, 50, 61, 117

houseleek, 17, 66, 89, 102, 121
hyssop, 28, 33, 50, 61, 116

indoor herb garden, 22-3
infusers, 49
insect-repellents, 33, 84-5
insomnia, 51, 80-1
itchy skin, 89

jasmine, 78, 80
juniper, 54, 63, 116

lanolin, 125
lavender, 20, 30, 36, 46, 50, 62, 63,
  66, 67, 72, 76, 80, 83, 102, 105,
  106, 117
lemon balm, 51, 56, 66, 118
lemon verbena, 19, 33, 51, 102,
  105, 117
limeflower tea, 51
liniments, 72
lip balm, lavender, 67
lovage, 11, 20, 21, 117

mace, 124
marigolds, 20, 21, 34, 68, 95, 114
marjoram, 11, 30, 74, 106, 119
medicinal herbs, 41-63
milk and honey bath oil, 90

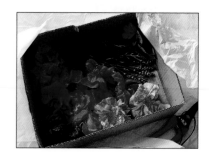